Examination and Surgical Skills OSCEs In Surgery

Jessamy Bagenal MBBS (Hons), BSc (Hons), MRCS

Kapil Sahnan MBBS (Hons), BSc (Hons), MRCS

Kaji Sritharan FRCS (Eng.), MD (Res.), FEBVS

© 2017 MD+ Publishing

I0042190

www.mrcspartbquestions.com

Published by: MD+ Publishing

Cover Design: Alexander Logan

ISBN-10: 0995662606

ISBN-13: 978-0995662605

Printed in the United Kingdom

CONTENTS

Contributors

Chapter 1: Examination

1.1 Cardiovascular 7
1.2 Respiratory 13
1.3 Lump A 16
1.4 Lump B 20
1.5 Abdominal A 24
1.6 Abdominal B 30
1.7 Groin Lump 35
1.8 Hernia 41
1.9 Stoma 46
1.10 Anterior Triangle 51
1.11. Neck Lump A 56
1.12 Neck Lump B 59
1.13 Posterior Triangle 62
1.14 Ear Discharge 66
1.15 Spine 70
1.16 Shoulder 78
1.17 Hand 84
1.18 Hip 93
1.19 Knee 100
1.20 Foot and Ankle 107
1.21 Cranial Nerve 114
1.22 Upper Limb Neurology 119
1.23 Lower Limb Neurology 124
1.24 Breast 127
1.25 Thyroid 132
1.26 Peripheral Vascular 136
1.27 Per Rectum 141
1.28 Testicular Exam 144
1.29 Ulcer 148
1.30 Varicose Veins 152

Chapter 2: Surgical Skills

2.1 Arterial Blood Gas 156
2.2 ATLS Survey 160
2.3 Blood Taking 163
2.4 Cannulation 165
2.5 Central Line 168
2.6 Chest Drain 171
2.7 Wound Debridement 175
2.8 Discharge/Transfer Summary. 178
2.9 Fine Needle Aspiration 180
2.10 Knee Joint Aspiration 183
2.11 Knot Tying. 187
2.12 Local Anaesthetic 190
2.13 Lumbar Puncture 193
2.14 Male Urethral Catheterisation 197
2.15 Needle Thoracostomy 201
2.16 Organising a List A 206
2.17 Organising a List B 212
2.18 Removal of a Naevus 218
2.19 Scrubbing Up 223
2.20 Suturing 226

MORE ONLINE

www.mrcspartbquestions.com

Access Over 1000 More MRCS Questions

Head over to the MRCS Part B website for our online MRCS Part B questions bank featuring over 1000 unique, interactive MRCS scenarios with comprehensive answers.

Created by high scoring, successful trainees the website and question bank can be accessed from your home computer, laptop or mobile device making your preparation as easy and convenient as possible.

Contributors

Stephen R Knight, BSc(Hons) MBChB(Hons) MRCS(Ed), Honorary Clinical Teacher University of Dundee, Perth Royal Infirmary, East of Scotland Deanery

Muhammed Alwahid, MBBS MRCS, Honorary Clinical Teacher University of Dundee, Perth Royal Infirmary, East of Scotland Deanery

Dr. Sari S Khaled MBBCh; Pinderfields Hospital; Yorkshire & Humber Deanery

Mr Ahmad S Khaled MBChB, MRCS; University College London Hospital; North Central Thames Deanery

Dr. Craig Goldsack BSc, MBChB, MRCP, FRCA; University College London Hospital; North Central Thames Deanery

Mr Graham Fulton BDS, MFDS RCPS, MBChB, MRCS University Hospital Southampton Wessex Deaney

Mr Madan Ethunandan BDS, MDS (OMFS), BM (Soton), MRCS (Edin), FRCS (OMFS), FDSRCS (Eng), FFDRCS (Irel) Consultant Oral and Maxillofacial Surgeon University Hospital Southampton Wessex Deanery

Charles Handford MBChB (Hons) MRCS General Duties Medical Officer The Royal Army Medical Corps, British Army.

Surgeon Commander Catherine Doran MD FRCS, Royal Navy Consultant Emergency and Colorectal Surgeon

Royal Navy Consultant Advisor in General Surgery The Queen Elizabeth Hospital, Birmingham

Mr. Ian Robertson BSc (Hons.) MBChB MRCS Medical Doctor and Core Surgical Trainee

Rachel Bowden MBChB MRCS Manchester University NHS Trust

1   EXAMINATION

1.1 Cardiovascular 7
1.2 Respiratory 13
1.3 Lump A 16
1.4 Lump B 20
1.5 Abdominal A 24
1.6 Abdominal B 30
1.7 Groin Lump 35
1.8 Hernia 41
1.9 Stoma. 46
1.10 Ear 51
1.11. Neck Lump A 56
1.12 Neck Lump B 59
1.13 Parotid Gland 62
1.14 Submandibular Swelling 66
1.15 Spine 70
1.16 Shoulder 78
1.17 Hand. 84
1.18 Hip 93
1.19 Knee. 100
1.20 Foot and Ankle 107
1.21 Cranial Nerve 114
1.22 Upper Limb Neurology 119
1.23 Lower Limb Neurology 124
1.24 Breast 127
1.25 Thyroid 132
1.26 Peripheral Vascular 136
1.27 Per Rectum. 141
1.28 Testicular Exam 144
1.29 Ulcer. 148
1.30 Varicose Veins 152

EXAMINATION

1.1 | Cardiovascular

Scenario

A 79-year-old retired solicitor will undergo an elective total hip replacement for osteoarthritis. He has come to see you in pre-operative assessment clinic.

The patient is comfortable, you have washed your hands, introduced yourself and explained what you are going to do. Please examine this patient's cardiovascular system and discuss and review any relevant investigations you wish to perform prior to surgery.

Describe how you would begin

Expose and inspect: Expose the patient's torso and legs. Have the patient sitting at 45 degrees on an examination couch.

ᏻ᠌ᡞ Findings

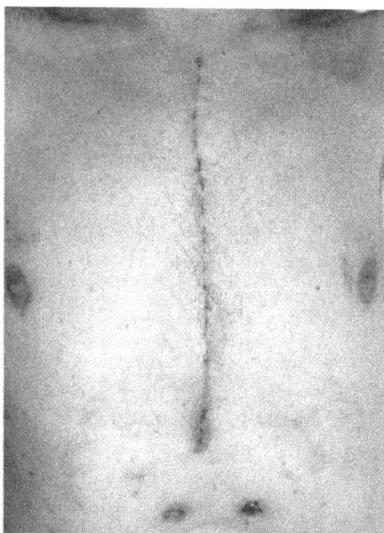

Describe what you see on inspection

On inspection there is a healed surgical incision of a median sternotomy.

Having inspected what would you do next?

Examine the cardiovascular system; pulse, BP, JVP, then focus on the precordium, palpation and auscultation, is there evidence of a pacemaker. Auscultate the lung bases. Examine the lower limbs, inspect for scars from vein harvesting, palpate for pulses, peripheral odema, and VTE, and assess the tissue viability in the feet.

> ### ⌒⌒ Findings
>
> This gentleman is comfortable at rest, he has a well-healed scar from a median sternotomy, and scars on the lower limbs consistent with vein harvesting for a coronary artery bypass graft. There are no stigmata of cardiac failure.

Differential diagnosis

Previous CABG
Valve replacement
Other mediastinal surgery

How will you manage the patient?

Full history (past medical, surgical and recent symptoms), and examination, notes review and review of any recent investigations. Explore the possible reasons the patient underwent cardiac surgery; ischemic heart disease, valvular disease and the sequelae of these such as atrial fibrillation and heart failure.

A thorough pre-operative work up is required. Request further investigations and an anaesthetic review.

What investigations are you going to request prior to surgery?

Patient specific:
Bloods: U&E, FBC, Coagulation, Group and Save
MRSA swabs
ECG – Looking for AF, cardiomegaly, right heart strain and any evidence of ischemia old/new
Chest Xray
Echocardiogram

Procedure specific:
Urine dip + MSU if dipstix +ve
Up to date AP pelvis and Lateral views of the side being operated on.

Blood tests and ECGs less than 3 months old do not routinely need repeating as long as there have been no changes in symptoms or medications and no new acute events during that time.

Formal face-to-face aesthetic review once results are available.

What will a transthoracic echocardiogram tell you?

A transthoracic echocardiogram will help detect and characterise coronary artery disease, will provide an indication of left and right ventricular function/dysfunction and significant arrhythmias.

It will also measure the ejection fraction, which if less than 50% is compatible with a diagnosis of systolic heart failure.

NB. A normal left ventricular ejection fraction does not exclude heart failure.

EXAMINATION

What are the benefits of good pre-operative assessment prior to elective surgery?

Safety – patients are risk assessed and investigated appropriately.
Ensures patient flow through the pathway from referral to surgery without undue delays, highlighting medical issues which need addressing / investigating prior to elective surgery. Reduces cancellation rates.

Do you know a system for grading patients?

The American Society of Anaesthetists grading system (ASA) grades patients according to their comorbidities to quantify the risk of mortality during and immediately post anaesthetic.

ASA 1- A normal healthy patient
ASA 2- A patient with mild systemic disease
ASA 3- A patient with severe systemic disease
ASA 4- A patient with severe systemic disease that is a constant threat to life
ASA 5- A moribund patient who is not expected to survive without the operation
ASA 6- A patient declared to be brain dead whose organs are being removed for donor purposes.

"E" added to the classification indicate emergency surgery.

What are the limitations of this system?

• Age is not taken into account.
• A patient with a single chronic stable disease scores the same as another with multiple.
• Definitions of a "systemic disease" are unclear
• It does not take into account the grade of surgery. (Grade 1 minor surgery – Grade 4 major surgery)

With all examinations first expose the patient, then inspect and examine before going on to comment on important additional points. Thank the patient, and offer the help them get dressed.

EXAMINATION SUMMARY

Pre-operative assessment is a way of risk assessing patients on a case by case basis. See NICE guielines on which investigations are required for which grade of surgery. Heart failure is a significant perioperative risk factor which if present doubles the risk of death after major surgery.

General Inspection

Look around bed for: medication, oxygen, insulin, chest leads, walking aids, medical-alert bracelet.
Does the patient look: well, breathless, well nourished. Any recognisable syndrome, how is the patient's complexion?

Exposure

Strip to the waist; 45 sitting upright
Use bed sheet to maintain patient's dignity while examining other systems.

EXAMINATION

Hands

Inspect dorsal and palmar aspects noting colour, skin texture, deformities and feel for temperature or sweating.
Fingers: tar-staining, finger clubbing, lipid deposits (xanthomata), palmar erythema, Dupryten's, Osler's nodes and Janeway lesions (Infective endocarditis).
Nails: koilonychias (spoon-shaped nail in iron deficiency), onycholysis (destruction), Beau's lines (chronic disease), Mee's lines (renal failure), Muehrcke's lines (hypoalbuminaemia), pitting (psoriasis/alopecia) and capillary nailbed pulsation (Quinke's sign of aortic regurge).

Pulse

Palpate the radial pulses and check for radial-radial delay and raise the arm up and feeling for collapsing pulse while gripping wrist.

Blood Pressure

Size the cuff and position the relaxed arm at the level of the heart
Inflate cuff till brachial pulse is occluded for maximum inflation pressure then deflate. Wait 15-20 seconds.
Listen with the diaphragm and inflate cuff then gradually deflate at rate of 2mmHg/second
Note B.P. to 2mmHg

Jugular Venous Pressure

Pt slightly looking to the left
Shine light/torch
Note cm above angle of Louis (normal =3cm)

Face

Eyes: Looking for anaemia, jaundice, corneal arcus, Kayser-Fleischer rings (Cu deposits, Wilson,s disease), xantholasma
Cheeks: Malar flush (mitral stenosis)
Mouth: Looking for central cyanosis, angular chelitis

Carotid pulse

Character & Volume: bounding pulses (CO2 retention, liver failure, sepsis), small volume (aortic stenosis, shock, pericardial effusions), collapsing (aortic incompetence, AV malformations, PDA), slow-rising (aortic stenosis), bisferiens (aortic stenosis+regurge), pulsus alternans (strong then weak - LVF, AS, cardiomyopathy), pulsus paradoxus (systolic weakens with inspiration - severe asthma, pericardial constriction, tamponade).

Thorax

Inspection
Praecordium for scars (look in apex) and ask patient to identify, implantable devices, colour, surface vessels, muscular deformity, breathing.
Assess capillary refill by pressing on the chest.

Palpation
Apex Beat: Hand below nipple feeling for maximal impulse then pinpoint midclavicular line 5th intercostal space and note the character.
Heave: palm on left sternal edge (thrusting pulsation indicating right ventricular enlargement).
Thrill: palm over aortic/pulmonary area (palpable murmur).

Auscultation

Place your finger on the carotid and listen at the mitral area (apex) with diaphragm and bell. Listen over the mitral area with the bell in left lateral position asking the patient to hold their breath to accentuate any murmurs.

Place the diaphragm over the tricuspid (5th IC left sternal edge), pulmonary (2nd IC left manubrial edge) and aortic (2nd IC right manubrial edge) areas.

Listen with the bell over the carotids.

Identify 1st and 2nd heart sounds, listen for added sounds and murmurs.

Murmurs

Inspiration accentuates right sided murmurs, expiration accentuates left sided murmurs.

Character: ejection-systolic (AS), pansystolic (MR), early-diastolic (AR), mid-diastolic (MS).

Radiation: ESM of AS radiate to carotids, PSM of MR to axilla.

Intensity: Graded systolic 1-6, diastolic 1-4.

1/6	Very soft
2/6	Soft but immediately detectable
3/6	Clearly audible, no thrill
4/6	Clearly audible, palpable thrill
5/6	Audible with stethoscope partially touching chest
6/6	Heard without stethoscope

Peripheral Pulses

Palpate popliteal (behind knee), posterior tibial (behind medial malleolus) and dorsalis pedis (1st/2nd metatarsals on anterior ankle) pulses.

Check for pitting oedema at feet and expose legs to look for vein harvest sites if you have not already done so.

References:

1. NICE guidance Preoperative tests for elective surgery. nice.org.uk/guidance/cg3
2. http://bestpractice.bmj.com/best-practice/monograph/954.html

TOP TIPS

➕ Pre-operative assessment is a common scenario in the MRCS OSCE examination. It is seen as a relatively straightforward station, but don't be lured into a false sense of security. Show the examiner you have a clear structure and work through it methodically.

➕ Whilst in reality an anaesthetic review might be sought you will be expected to review and comment upon investigation results such as an ecg, be systematic in your approach to interpreting these *(rate, rhythm, etc).*

➕ Be cautious not to just reel off a list of tests and investigations without having good reasoning for doing them.

EXAMINATION

1.2 | Respiratory

Scenario

A 62 year old gentleman is referred to the surgical pre-assessment clinic for a right-sided elective inguinal hernia repair. The patient is comfortable, you have washed you hands, introduced yourself and explained what you are going to do. Please take a brief history, examine him as appropriate and discuss your findings with the examiner.

Describe how you would begin

As the title suggests, this is a pre-assessment clinic and you would not be expected to examine in any detail the hernia itself. First begin by introducing yourself and confirming that he has a hernia awaiting repair you should start with a quick but comprehensive medical and surgical history. A good starting question might be, "What other medical conditions do you have?"

> ### History findings
> This gentleman is comfortable at rest, he has a well-healed scar from a median sternotomy, and scars on the lower limbs consistent with vein harvesting for a coronary artery bypass graft. There are no stigmata of cardiac failure.

You find that he has COPD and has been a life-long smoker with an approximate 30 pack year exposure. He has difficulty walking up more than one flight of stairs and takes two inhalers for this.

What further questions might be useful at this point?

It would be worthwhile finding out how well his COPD is controlled, how often he uses his short-acting reliever inhaler and if he has regular chest infections. You could also ask if he has ever needed to be referred to a respiratory physician or been admitted to hospital with his COPD.

You might also like to ask about his cardiovascular and performance status.

> ### ᏼᏒ Further history
> He denies any cardiac symptoms of angina or ankle swelling but is a controlled hypertensive on Amlodipine. He also takes a statin. He is not on home oxygen.

Having taken a history what would you do next?

You should then proceed to examine his respiratory system beginning with an inspection of his overall state.

EXAMINATION

After inspection what comes next?

You should start with his nails examining for clubbing, look for a hypercapnic flap and palpate for a bounding pulse.

You should then examine the face checking for signs of cyanosis or anaemia before moving onto inspection, palpation, auscultation and percussion of his chest.

Palpation, ausculatation and percussion

Palpate the trachea, looking for signs of deviation or tracheal tug. Chest expansion should be performed with both hands at the same time on the anterior chest and then posteriorly for lateral movement.

Perform auscultation and percussion side-to-side for comparison and over the entirety of the lung fields. Sit the patient up and repeat at the back where signs of basal crepitations (heart failure) will be most evident.

> ### ⌒ Findings
>
> Examination On inspection, he has a large body habitus and pursed lips when breathing. He has a barrel-shaped hyper-expanded chest and his breathing has a prolonged expiratory phase with mild end-expiratory wheeze. There are no further findings.

Is there anything else you would like to do?

Offer to examine the abdomen for any previous surgery and examine the hernia to check that it is an inguinal hernia which is reducible and non-tender. You might also ask for some formal observations such as blood pressure, pulse rate, respiratory rate and saturations.

Please summarise your findings

This station will simply require a summary of your main findings as the diagnosis has already been made for you.

How will you manage the patient?

This patient will require a pre-operative lung function test, echocardiogram, chest X-ray, ECG and blood tests (FBC, LFTs, U+Es). The type of hernia repair he undergoes will be dependent on the results. For instance, it is unlikely he will be able to undergo a laparoscopic hernia repair.

What would you expect to find from the lung function tests for this gentleman?

The main test would be spirometry, which measures the volume of air exhaled during forceful exhalation. You would expect an "obstructive" picture evident within the lung function tests, which is a decreased FEV1/FVC (Forced Expiratory Volume over 1 second/ Forced Vital Capacity) ratio as well as a decreased FEV1. These are compared to predicted values taking into account their weight and height. Normal or raised FEV1/FVC ratios on the other hand would suggest a restrictive pathology.

EXAMINATION

Findings

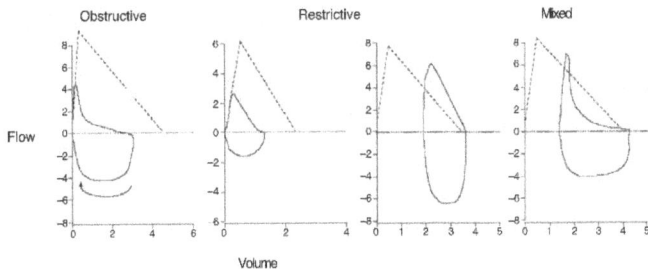

What are you looking for with the echocardiogram?

Together with the ECG you are looking for signs of right heart strain (cor pulmonale) indicating severe disease. This is exhibited by right bundle branch block and/or right axis deviation on the ECG and pulmonary hypertension with associated right ventricular hypertrophy/dilatation on echo.

How would you manage a patient with severe COPD?

As with all decisions in surgery, an assessment of risks vs. benefits must be made together with the patient. Severe or poorly managed COPD is not an absolute contraindication but will increase the risk of postoperative pulmonary complications such as atelectasis, pneumonia, and perhaps prolonged post-operative mechanical ventilation within an HDU/ITU environment. If this is detected early and surgery can wait, lifestyle modification including smoking cessation and best medical therapy will improve their fitness for theatre. This patient will probably be more suitable for a hernia repair under local anesthetic

Who else might you discuss your findings with?

Close liaison with anaesthetic colleagues in the run-up to the operation means that these risks can be anticipated and potentially avoided and will be necessary if a post-operative HDU bed is necessary for weaning off ventilation. Involvement of a respiratory physician might be helpful if you have an uncertain diagnosis or are worried about poor control.

TOP TIPS

Although this specific scenario covers both history-taking and examination, be sure to read the briefing carefully in case the exam wants you to focus mainly on one or the other. Practise both versions. You may need to take a full history and only offer to examine the patient, or you may need to perform an examination only, which may cover both respiratory and cardiovascular systems. The key will be practising within the time limits given.

EXAMINATION

1.3 | Lump A

Scenario

A 73 year old retired serviceman attends your lumps and bumps clinic with a raised, slow growing lesion on the dorsum of his hand

The patient is comfortable, you have washed your hands, introduced yourself and explained what you are going to do. Please examine this lump

Describe how you would begin

Expose and Inspect: Expose both upper limbs to the shoulder Sit the patient opposite you on a chair with their hands resting on a pillow.

Inspect the lump thoroughly before looking for any additional lesions or scars from previous surgery. Also take note of the patients skin type, as well as any areas of hyperpigmentation.

Note: If a skin lesion is suspected, pay particular attention to other areas of sun exposure: the face, scalp, neck, shoulders, arms and lower legs.

Inspection Findings

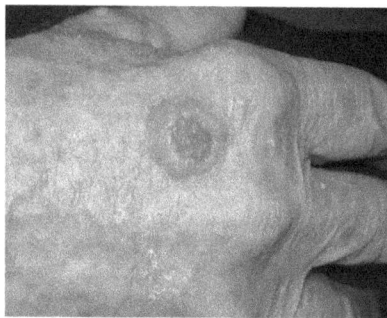

Describe what you see on inspection

On inspection there is a raised lesion on the dorsum of the hand measuring approximately 1.5cm diameter. The lesion is pink in colour with pearly rolled edges, a central ulcerated core and telangiectasia.

Having inspected what would you do next?

Palpation
Palpate the lump for temperature, size, shape, edges, consistency, fluctance and fixity to underlying structures.

Additional examination
Remember to examine the axilla for lymph nodes

You should also examine the neurovascular status of the limb as very occasionally there

EXAMINATION

may be invasion of underlying deeper structures.

> #### ⌒ Findings
>
> The lump has a raised pearly edge, with a crusty central core, which bleeds
> easily. There is no fixation to underlying structures. The gentleman has a fair skin
> type with evidence of previous significant sun exposure.

Differential diagnosis

- Epidermis – Basal cell carcinoma, Squamous Cell Carcinoma, Malignant melanoma,
  Keratoacanthoma
- Subcutaneous – lipoma, fibroma

Are you aware of any pre-malignant skin conditions?

Actinic keratosis (Solar/senile keratosis) – A premalignant thickening of the epidermis,
with associated redness and scale. This condition represents dysplastic change with no
invasion of the basal layer.
Bowen's disease – when there is dysplastic change invading the basal layer
Both Actinic keratosis and Bowen's disease may progress to squamous cell carcinoma

What is the likely diagnosis

Basal Cell Carcinoma. The most common skin cancer in the Europe, Australia and the
U.S.A. The incidence of BCC is increasing worldwide. (1) Particularly affecting elderly
males, although cases in adults as young as 40 with significant sun exposure have been
reported.

What risk factors predispose to the development of this condition?

Genetic predisposition
Exposure to ultraviolet radiation
Fair skin types
Immunosuppression
Male sex

How will you manage the patient?

Conservative
Conservative measures include offering advice on sun exposure
Management of low-risk superficial skin lesions depends upon the size and location of the
lesion.

Medical
Small superficial lesions may be managed with regular application of topical immune
stimulating agents e.g. Imiquimod

Surgical
Larger lesions are likely to require excision biopsy.
Lesions in cosmetically sensitive areas may be excised using Mohs micrographically
controlled exesion techniques.
Lesions around the eye may require referral to specialist oculoplastic centres.

Can you summarise the layers of the skin

The skin may be divided into 3 layers. Epidermis, Dermis and Subcutis

EXAMINATION

The epidermis may be subdivided into 3 further layers – Stratum corneum, Stratum Spinosum, Stratum Basale

Dermis – Containing a mixture of tissue types: Sebaceous glands, sweat glands, neural cells, papillary muscle, and blood vessels

Subcutis – Consists primarily of fat and blood vessels

With reference to Malignant melanoma, what staging systems are you aware of

Breslow's Thickness

A system used to stage melanoma based on its depth of invasion measured in millimeters. Stages extend from stage 1 to 5. (2) Breslow staging may be use to prognosticate approximate 5 year survival and risk of metastasis. This system was originally described by Alexander Breslow in 1970, but has now largely been superseded by the TMN system, where T 'Primary tumour' includes depth of invasion.

What do you understand about Mohs micrographically controlled excision?

Mohs Micrographic surgery is a technique employed for the excision of lesions in cosmetically sensitive locations (face, eyes, lips, nose), or ill-defined BCCs. Using a microtome, thin layers of skin are successively removed and examined for histology under a microscope during the operation. The microtome excisions continue until there is no further histological extension of the tumour. This technique aims to spare as much healthy tissue as possible, limiting the cosmetic implications whilst minimising the risk of recurrence.

EXAMINATION

EXAMINATION SUMMARY

With all potentially malignant skin conditions first expose the patient, then inspect the lesion itself before going on to comment on important additional points such as skin type, other lesions and scars. Examine the lesion systematically starting with simple palpation, before going on to test for fixity/fluctuance etc. Take care to examine the relevant lymphatic drainage site(s). Thank the patient, and offer the help them get dressed.

TOP TIPS

➕ Lumps and bumps come up frequently in the MRCS OSCE examination. It is seen as a relatively straightforward station, but don't be lured into a false sense of security. Show the examiner you have a clear structure and work through this methodically.

➕ Demonstrate knowledge by commenting on the patients skin type, examining for lymphadenopathy and looking for other lesions particularly in sun-exposed sites.

References:

1. Telfer NR, Colver GB, Morton C a. Guidelines for the management of basal cell carcinoma. Br J Dermatol. 2008;159(1):35–48.
2. Breslow A. Thickness, cross-sectional areas and depth of invasion in the prognosis of cutaneous melanoma. Ann Surg [Internet]. 1970 Nov [cited 2015 Apr 19];172(5):902–8. Available from: http://www.pubmedcentral.nih.gov/articlerender.fcgi?artid=1397358&tool=pmcentrez&rendertype=abstract
3. Clark WH, Elder DE, Guerry D, Braitman LE, Trock BJ, Schultz D, et al. Model predicting survival in stage I melanoma based on tumor progression. J Natl Cancer Inst [Internet]. 1989 Dec 20 [cited 2015 Sep 6];81(24):1893–904. Available from: http://www.ncbi.nlm.nih.gov/pubmed/2593166

EXAMINATION

1.4 | Lump B

Scenario

A 42 year old accountant attends your lumps and bumps clinic with a painless lump on his back that has been there for many years.

The patient is comfortable, you have washed your hands, introduced yourself and explained what you are going to do. Please examine the lump

Describe how you would begin

Expose and Inspect: Fully expose the area of the lump and the surrounding skin.

Inspect the lump thoroughly. Identifiy the location of the lump in respect to surrounding anatomy. Inspect the size and shape of the lump, making note of colour and any skin changes.

Look for scars suggestive of previous surgery.

Ask the patient if there are any similar lumps elsewhere.

Inspection Findings

Describe what you see on inspection

On inspection there is a 4cm hemispherical swelling over the medial aspect of the left scapular. There are no visible skin changes.

Having inspected what would you do next?

Palpation
Check whether the lump is tender beforehand.
Palpate the lump for size, shape and whether the edges are well or poorly defined. Assess consistency (is it soft or hard?) and note any temperature changes. Asses whether the lump is mobile or attached to underlying structures.

EXAMINATION

Try to ascertain which plain the lump is in by attempting to move the skin over the lump and palpating the lump when the underlying muscle is both contracted and relaxed.

> ### ᕦ Findings
> The lump is soft, non-tender and has a lobulated surface. The skin moves freely over the top of it. It exhibits the 'slip sign' i.e. it slips away on gentle touch.

Differential diagnosis

- Epidermis – Epidermal cyst
- Subcutaneous – lipoma, fibroma, liposarcoma, abscess, haematoma

Given the location and consistency of this lump, it is likely to be a lipoma. Since the patient has had this for many years and there is no suggestion of any changes in size it is unlikely this is a liposarcoma.

How will you manage this patient?

Conservative
Watch and wait if asymptomatic.

Surgical
- Smaller lipomas can generally be excised under local anaesthetic. An incision is made over the top of the lipoma and attempts are made to remove the lipoma as a whole.
- Liposuction can be used if the lipoma is soft and there is concern about scarring. However, it may fail to remove the entire mass, making recurrence more likely.
- Corticosteroid injections may also be used in small lipomas to induce lypolisis and shrink the lipoma. However, since the lipoma is not fully removed, recurrence is highly likely.

What is this similar skin lesion?

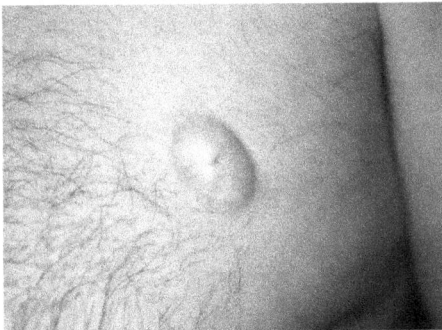

This is an epidermal (formerly sebaceous) cyst. To differentiate between the two, look for the central hole (punctum) present in epidermal cysts. Cysts tend to be firmer and closer to the surface

What is the difference between an epidermal cyst and a lipoma?

Epidermal cysts are filled with keratin and lined with stratified squamous epithelium. The

EXAMINATION

term 'sebaceous cyst' is a misnomer as the cysts are not components of sebaceous glands and are not filled with sebum. Lipomas are comprised of adipocytes.

Do lipomas have malignant potential?

There is currently no evidence that lipomas undergo malignant change and people with lipomas are not more likely to develop liposarcomas.

What are liposarcomas?

Liposarocomas are rare lipomatous tumours, which typically occur in middle aged and older people in the lower limb (they can however arise anywhere). They can be difficult to differentiate from lipomas, particularly when they are slow growing.

How are liposarcomas classified?

They can be classified into 4 biological groups: well-differentiated, dedifferentiated, myxoid / round cell and pleomorphic.

Do you know of any syndromes associated with lipomas?

Adiposis Dolorosa (Dercum's disease) – a rare condition characterised by multiple painful lipomas.

Bannayan-Zonana syndrome – a rare inherited disease involving multiple lipomas, marcocephaly and haemangiomas.

EXAMINATION SUMMARY

Wash hands
Introduce, gain consent and expose patient – ensure that you adequately expose the lump and any surrounding skin

Inspect – make a mental note of the size and location of the lump, along with its relationship with surrounding structures. Look at the surrounding skin for any changes.

Palpate – systematically examine the lump, feeling for size, consistency (is it fluctuant/ firm etc.), mobility. Try and elicit which layer the lump is in.

Closing – Thank the patient and inform them they can now get dressed. Present your findings.

References:
1. Luba MC, Bangs SA, Mohler AM, Stulberg DL. Common benign skin tumors. Am Fam Physician. 2003 Feb 15;67(4):729-38.
2. Dalal KM1, Antonescu CR, Singer S. Diagnosis and management of lipomatous tumors. J Surg Oncol. 2008 Mar 15;97(4):298-313.

TOP TIPS

➕ Ensure you have a good understanding of the different benign skin lumps and how they feel as this will allow you to differentiate between them in the exam. When talking about management of benign skin lumps don't forget that your first answer should be conservative and expectant management if the lump is not causing the patient problems. Be systematic in your approach to this examination to demonstrate to the examiner that you have a clear structure.

EXAMINATION

1.5 | Abdominal A

Scenario

A 20-year-old female presents with a 24-hour history of abdominal pain that was initially generalised but is now in the RIF. She is nauseated and anorexic. She has no previous significant medical or surgical history and is normally well.

Although the patient has a level of underlying pain she is comfortable enough to be examined. You have washed your hands, introduced yourself and explained what you are going to do. Please perform an appropriate abdominal examination.

Describe how you would begin

Expose, position and inspect: Expose the patient from the nipple line to the groin crease (note that the classical 'nipple to knee' is no longer appropriate or necessary unless later findings warrant further groin/genital examination). Ask the patient to lie fully supine if possible. Remember not to just inspect the patient but also look for stigmata around the bedside.

🔍 Findings

The patient is alert and orientated. There are no abdominal scars. She has a peripheral venous cannula in her right antecubital fossa with a bag of Hartmans solution running. There is an empty vomit bowel next to the bed, her breath is ketotic. Her observations reveal a tympanic membrane temperature of 38.2 °C, she is normotensive and has a heart rate of 110bpm. When you lay her flat the movement worsened her pain.

Describe what you see on inspection

Concise communication of the key positives and poignant negatives will impress the examiner. This can be done at the end of the exam or following end of bed inspection.

Describe what you would do next

Peripheral examination: This involves a systematic examination starting in the hands, working up to the neck, then the face and inspecting the thorax. Examples of relevant findings for each area are as follows (non exhaustive list):

Hands: Capillary refill, nail changes.
Wrist: Radial pulse rate.
Face: Evidence of anaemia when the inner eyelid is inspected, angular stomatitis, glossitis.
Neck: Lymphadenopathy noting Virchow's node.
Thorax: Laboured/rapid respiration.

Abdominal examination: Focus on the abdomen after a systematic generalised examination. This begins with close inspection; remember that scars can often be difficult to see if in skin creases. At this point it is useful to ask the patient to cough or lift their head off the bed, this may reveal hernias or a divarication of the recti and also gives an indication as to whether the patient is peritonitic.

Begin palpating. Ensure your arm and shoulder are at the same level as the patients abdomen, kneeling may make this easier. Ask the patient again to state where their pain is and warn them you are about to palpate their abdomen. Palpate systematically and start away from the area of pain, in this case starting in the LIF would be sensible. Palpate all 9 regions. Initial palpation is soft followed by deep palpation. Observe the patients face throughout for signs of discomfort.

Look for organomegaly after general palpation. This includes balloting the kidneys, palpating for the spleen and the liver. In this case do not start in the RIF when palpating for the spleen/liver as this will cause unnecessary pain. Next percuss and assess the size of the spleen and the liver.

To finish the examination, palpate for a palpable expansile abdominal aorta, auscultate for bowel sounds and perform any special tests (Rosvings sign/ Obturator sign/Psoas sign). It is also good practice to expose the lower legs to assess for oedema or, admittedly rare, extra gastro-intestinal signs such as pyoderma gangrenosum, which can be indicative of inflammatory bowel disease and is a cause of RIF pain.

> ### ⟨⟩ Findings
> The patient has a dry tongue, a strong but fast radial pulse. There are no stigmata of chronic disease. Examination of the abdomen reveals localized peritonism over the RIF and Rosvings sign is positive. No organomegally is found.

How would you end the examination?

Thank the patient, cover them up and turn to the examiner. Place your hands behind your back and say how you would like to finish your examination. Consider stating you would like to examine for inguinal hernias, perform a digital rectal examination (DRE) and examine the external genitalia. Remember if you are going to state you would do any of these always mention you would ensure there is a chaperone present and be able to clinically justify them. The findings must therefore aid your diagnosis or alter your management plan. A DRE should not be considered a routine/indicated examination if you are suspecting appendicitis[1].

At this point of the station it is worth mentioning the need for urinalysis and urinary beta-HCG. Although a simple bedside test rather than examination it will highlight to the examiner that you are already thinking logically to exclude key differentials.

Present your findings

Ensure this is concise and includes your positive findings and relevant negative findings.

What is your differential diagnosis?

Be systematic in presenting your differential, however present the most likely diagnosis first and be prepared to justify your differentials.

Gastrointestinal: Acute appendicitis, inflamed Meckel's diverticulum, inflammatory bowel disease, bowel cancer, caecal volvulus, inguinal hernia, viral gastritis, cholecystitis, mysenteric lymphadenopathy/adentitis (more common in adolescents and paediatrics[2]), non-specific abdominal pain.

Urological: Urinary tract infection, renal colic, pyelonephritis.

EXAMINATION

Gynaecological: Ectopic pregnancy, pelvic inflammatory disease, ovarian cyst/torsion, ruptured Graafian follicle (mittelschmerz).

Vascular: Dissecting aortic/iliac aneurysm.

Musculoskeletal: Psoas abscess, rectus sheath haematoma.

In this case assuming the patients' beta HCG is negative appendicitis or gynaecological pathology is most likely.

What is your immediate management?

Start with an ABCDE assessment with review of available observations and any pre-existing clerking. Once happy the patient is stable they should be placed nil by mouth and started on intravenous fluids. Analgesia titrated to pain and anti-emetics should be prescribed, paracetamol is beneficial as both an analgesic and anti-pyretic. If the patient is acutely unwell titrated oxygen therapy may also be warranted.

What tests and investigations would you organise for a differential diagnosis of appendicitis?

Urinalysis and beta HCG. Remember not to be mislead by positive leucocyte and blood readings as this can be associated with a pelvic or retrocaecal lying appendix.

Blood tests. Full blood count, urea and electrolytes, C-reactive protein, clotting studies and a group and save should be obtained.

Venous blood gas with attention to lactate.

Blood culture if pyrexial.

Cusco speculum examination when indicated by patient history and symptoms (e.g. suspicion of PID), but only if a chaperone is present and you have access to the appropriate swab containers.

Ultrasonography is used in female patients to exclude gynaecological pathology. It can at times visualise the appendix but it is limited in its diagnostic ability in acute appendicitis and if normal cannot exclude appendicitis therefore it is performed to help exclude a gynecological cause[3].

Computer tomography (CT) has now become common practice as first line imaging in the investigation of abdominal pain suggestive of appendicitis in patients over the age of 50[4].

Magnetic resonance imaging (MRI) is used as an alternative to CT in the pregnant patient and is highly sensitive[5].

Diagnostic laparoscopy. Remember this is invasive and appropriate consent and risk benefit analysis must be undertaken; ensure you consent for what you will do upon discovery of pathology.

Remember in the acutely unwell patient do not delay an operative procedure while awaiting for tests or for their results as acute appendicitis can be a clinical diagnosis.

What are your treatment options?

Conservative/medical: Traditionally only undertaken if surgery unavailable (i.e. in a remote setting) or if the patient is unfit for surgery. This involves a course of antibiotics and observation. However be aware for your exam that there is growing evidence for treating uncomplicated appendicitis with a course of antibiotics rather than surgery[6][7].

Surgical: Laparoscopic appendectomy is the preferred option in many centres, however there are cases where open appendectomy is performed[8].

If during an appendicectomy the appendix appears normal which other structures should routinely be sought for/viewed?

Trace two feet of distal small bowel for a Meckel's Diverticulum which can cause similar symptoms to appendicitis. View the pelvis thoroughly in female patients examining the ovaries and uterus for signs of PID or endometriosis alongside visualization of both ovaries.

There is no consensus on whether a macroscopically normal appendix should be removed or left in situ. Some argue that a macroscopically normal appendix can be found to show histological pathology and thus opt for removal in the absence of finding a causative pathology in the abdomen/pelvis for the patients symptoms[9][10]. However others argue one should leave the macroscopically normal appendix in situ as removal is associated with risk and increases patient morbidity compared to that of diagnostic laparoscopy alone[11][12].

Describe the anatomical layers one would encounter when approaching the appendix during open removal?

Skin
Campers' fascia
Scarpa's fascia
External oblique
Internal oblique
Transversus abdominis
Transverse fascia
Preperitoneal fat
Parietal peritoneum

Discuss the principles behind laparoscopic port site placement during an appendectomy?

The concept of port triangulation must be followed. Typically a port for the camera is placed at the umbilicus, then two further ports are placed to form a triangle. These ports can be located in the RLQ/LLQ/RUQ or suprapupic region and this is down to the discretion of the surgeon[13]. Remember that increasingly minimal techniques utilizing two ports or a single port are being used.

How would you insert your ports?

I would insert the first port using the open Hassan technique and then the following ports under direct visualization.

During laparoscopic appendectomy you discover a perforated appendix with pus contaminating the peritoneal cavity, how would you manage this?

At this point one has to decide if a conversion to an open procedure is required. If there is four-quadrant contamination it may be appropriate to perform a lower midline incision to ensure safe removal of the appendix and full washout. Some would advocate performing a thorough wash out laparoscopically before converting to open to remove the appendix.

Some may opt to manage a perforation with contamination laparoscopically and I will now discuss how this is done. Firstly the appendix must be removed and appendicular stump closed. When the appendix is delivered it must be through the port and not touch the tissue of the abdominal wall to help minimize infection risk. Next suction purulent fluid and attempt to locate any faecoliths. Perform generous irrigation, irrigating the entire peritoneal cavity, changing the tilt of the operating table can be useful in ensure this. Once the irrigating fluid has been removed and there is no obvious visible contamination the ports can be removed with a drain left in the RIF[14][15].

Post operatively the patient must be started on a course of antibiotics (initially intravenous) and monitored for signs of sepsis and subsequent abdominal collection.

Why does the classical pain of appendicitis move from the umbilicus to the RIF?

In early appendicitis pain is carried via the autonomic nervous system due to irritation of the visceral peritoneum, this is known as visceral pain. This is poorly located and follows embryological origins, the appendix is a midgut structure so pain is felt in the umbilical region.

As the appendicitis progresses the parietal peritoneum is irritated. The parietal peritoneum is innervated by the somatic nervous system so the pain is more easily localised. This is known as somatic pain.

SUMMARY OF EXAMINATION

Introduce
Intorduce and explain that you are going to examine the abdomen.
Exposure: Nipples to knees (in practice use a sheet to cover external genitalia and maintain dignity.)
Position: Lower bed flat, with patient resting on one pillow. Arms by sides.

Inspect
Distension, scars. drains and stomas (follow the drain and see what is draining and identify the type of stoma), masses, vessels, striae, hernias.
Ask the patient to raise their head off the pillow, breathe in and out, suck their tummy and give a cough. As they do this look for herniae and diversification of the herniae.

Palpation & Percussion
Assess for a triple A by placing hands either side of the umbilicus.
Feel for hernias in the inguinal region and ask patient to cough.
Squat by side of bed so patient's abdomen is at eye level.
Look at the patient's face and begin light palpation at the point farthest from pain. Palpate in four quadrants. Once your have palpated lightly repeat pressing more firmly.
If you suspect any herniae ask the patient to cough and follow the detailed hernia exam detailed later in the text.
Palpating a mass: feel for size, shape, surface, consistency, mobility, pulsatile nature, movement with respiration.

Liver: begin in the right iliac fossa, exert gentle pressure and ask the patient to breathe in

EXAMINATION

and out. With inspiration drift your palm upwards towards the liver.
Percuss the liver – map out the upper and lower borders of liver by sequential plapation.
Map out the top from the resonant lung field and then the bottom of liver from the right lower quadrant.
Normal: Around 5th IC midline to costal margin.

Spleen: begin in the right iliac fossa below the umbilicus. Ask the patient to breathe in and out moving towards the left costal margin.
Percuss the Spleen - percuss from the umbilicus to the left costal margin.

Kidneys: Place your left hand behind the right loin. Place your right hand at the costal margin. Push down with your right hand balloting the kidney. Repeat for the left kidney.

Percussion
Ascites – Percuss centrally, from the umbilicus to the flank on the left side. Ask the patient to roll towards you and percuss their back if ascites present.

Auscultate
Listen for 15-20 seconds for bowel sounds
Listen for renal bruits – press down firmly a few cm above the umbilicus at the lateral edge of the rectus muscle.
Listen for femoral bruits over the femoral pulse.

State to Examiners
That you would examine the external genitalia, dipstick the urine and perform a PR examination.

EXAMINATION

TOP TIPS

✚ Never forget a pregnancy test and gynecological causes of abdominal pain in the female patient.

✚ Always avoid causing the patient unnecessary pain. For example in this case examining for shifting dullness would cause pain and is unlikely to provide clinical benefit.

✚ If an elderly patient presents with iliac fossa pain ensure you feel for an abdominal aneurysm.

1.6 | Abominal B

Scenario

A 65-year-old male presents with a gradual history of an increasingly distended abdomen, generalized weight loss and his wife has told him he looks yellow despite no recent holiday. The patient is comfortable. You have washed your hands, introduced yourself and explained what you are going to do. Please examine this gentleman's abdomen.

Describe how you would begin

Expose, position and inspect: Expose the patient from the nipple line to the groin crease (note that the classical 'nipple to knee' is no longer appropriate or necessary unless later findings warrant further groin/genital examination). Remember in all situations where a patient is exposed, especially if down to underwear, dignity must be maintained, only expose when necessary and give the patient a blanket to maintain their modesty when exposure is not needed. Chaperones must be used when indicated. Ask the patient to lie fully supine if possible. Remember not to just inspect the patient but also look for stigmata around the bedside.

Describe what you see on inspection

Concise communication of the key positives and poignant negatives will impress the examiner. This can be done at the end of the exam or following end of bed inspection.

Findings

The patient is alert, orientated and comfortable. There are no abdominal scars or tattoos. He is mildly distended and cachectic in the upper body. He appears jaundiced with evidence of mild excoriation.

Describe what you would do next

Peripheral examination: This involves a systematic examination starting with the hands, working up to the neck, then the face, inspecting the thorax and feeling for sacral edema. Example of relevant findings for each area are as follows (non exhaustive list):

Hands: Nail changes, palmar erethema, wasting
Wrist: Radial pulse, Asterixis (liver flap), 'track marks'
Face: Jaundice, angular stomatitis, glossitis
Neck: Lymphadenopathy noting Virchow's node, raised JVP
Thorax: Spider naevi, gynaecomastia in the male patient

Abdominal examination: Now focus on the abdomen itself. Begin with close inspection; remember that scars can often be difficult to see if in skin creases. At this point it is useful to ask the patient to cough or with the patient flat keeping their shoulders on the bed ask them to raise their head to look at their feet. This may reveal hernias/divarification of recti and also give an indication as to whether the patient is peritonitic or not.

Palpation. At this point re-ascertain with the patient that they are not in pain and warn them that you are about to start palpating their abdomen and kneel next to the patient. Palpate systematically with all 9 regions palpated. Initial palpation is soft followed by deep palpation.

Look for organomegaly. This includes balloting the kidneys. Palpate for the spleen and the liver starting from the RIF timed to breathing. Also percuss the liver from above assessing for inferior displacement. Following this percuss out the borders of the spleen. At this point the bladder can also be percussed.

Feel for an abdominal aorta, although this is unlikely to be felt on a background of distension.

Auscultate for bowel sounds.

Test for ascites, this is classically done in one off two ways, either testing for shifting dullness or a fluid thrill.

At the end of the examination it is useful to expose the lower leg to assess if there is peripheral edema, if the patient has been lying for a prolonged period sacral oedema may be a better marker.

👓 Findings

The patient is cachectic. He has palmar erythema and spider naevi on the thorax. He is jaundiced with shifting dullness present. He has a large irregular palpable liver edge. There is no asterixis.

EXAMINATION

How would you end the examination?

Thank the patient and turn around to the examiner. Place your hands behind your back and say how you would like to finish your examination. *'To complete my examination I would like to palpate for inguinal hernias, examine the external genitalia and perform a digital rectal examination.'* Remember if you state you wish to perform these more intrusive areas of examination you must be able to justify them and have a chaperone present.

Present your findings.

Ensure this is concise and includes your positive findings and relevant negative findings.

What causes of hepatomegaly do you know?

As always attempt to structure your answer with a surgical sieve.

Neoplastic: Primary vs secondary
Infective: Hepatitis, Epstein-Barr virus, Malaria
Immunological: Primary sclerosing cholangitis
Inflammatory: Cirrhotic (early)
Metabolic: Amyloidosis, haemochromatosis
Vascular: Budd-Chiari syndrome, right sided heart failure
Iatrogenic: Methotrexate
Environmental: Alcohol excess, Non-alcoholic fatty liver disease

What is your differential diagnosis specific for this case?

The patient is elderly presenting with liver failure and a palpable irregular hepatomegaly, the likely potential causes relevant for this case include;

Neoplastic: Primary (e.g. hepatocellular) vs metastatic (e.g. colorectal)
Infective: Hepatitis (chronic or acute)
Environmental: Alcohol excess
Immunological: Primary sclerosing cholangitis (always ask about a history of IBD in these patients)

What would your short-term (i.e first 48 hours) management of this patient consist of?

After initial ABCDE assessment and review of the observation chart to confirm the patient is stable I would implement the following.

Treatment:

Analgesia as required: Beware opiate accumulation in liver failure.

Laxatives: In all patients with liver failure regular daily bowel movements help prevent encephalopathy.

Nutritional supplementation: If available involve the dietician team.

Antibiotics: If signs of spontaneous bacterial peritonitis.

Investigations:

Bloods and peripheral venous access: These must include the usual FBC, U&S's, LFT's and clotting screens. Consider tumour markers such as CEA. Send a liver screening panel. If pyrexic perform blood cultures.

Note: In ascitic patients hold off intra-venous fluids unless strong indication.

Abdominal radiograph: Ensuring there is no evidence of underlying bowel obstruction causing distension.

Ascitic tap/drain: Send for MC&S and cytology. If signs of spontaneous bacterial peritonitis do not delay intravenous antibiotics. This is a test with the additional benefit of temporary therapeutic relief if a drain is left in situ.

Computer Tomography: In this case liver metastasis is a likely potential cause. He will need imaging of his thorax, abdomen and pelvis with contrast.

Refer for discussion at a multi-disciplinary team meeting.

Describe the normal surface anatomy of the liver.

The superior marking is from along the nipple line relating to the 5th rib. Lateral makings are the thoracic wall on the right side and the left midclavicular line. Inferiorly the liver is marked by the right costal margin. This makes a triangular structure.

Which cancers commonly metastasise to the Liver?

Colorectal

EXAMINATION

Bronchial
Breast
Ovarian
Melanoma
Pancreatic
Cholangiocarcinoma

Can you tell me ways in which cancer can spread?

Direct invasion
Haematogenous
Lymphatic
Transcoelomic
Iatrogenic seeding

What types of jaundice do you know?

Jaundice can be classified into pre-hepatic, hepatic and post hepatic jaundice. These can be deduced by looking at the colour of the patients stool and urine alongside reviewing the patients liver function tests.

	Pre-Hepatic	Hepatic	Post-Hepatic
Urine colour	Normal		
Dark	Dark		
Stool colour	Normal	Normal	Pale
AST	Normal	Very High	Normal/High
ALP	Normal	Normal/High	Very High
Bilirubin	High	High	High

How can ascites be classified?

Ascites classically has been classified as transudate or exudate depending on its protein content, transudate having a low protein content and exudate being high. However a better measure is the serum-ascites albumin gradient (SAAG)[1][2]. A high gradient is >1.1 g/dL while a low gradient is <1.1 g/dL. A high gradient is in keeping with transudate and a low with exudate.

SAAG Gradient	
>1.1 g/dL	<1.1 g/dL
Portal Hypertension	Peritoneal infection (i.e TB)
Hypoproteinaemia	Peritoneal carcinomatosis
Liver metastasis/neoplasia	Pancreatitis
Cirrhosis	

EXAMINATION

SUMMARY OF EXAMINATION

Introduce
Intorduce and explain that you are going to examine the abdomen.
Exposure: Nipples to knees (in practice use a sheet to cover external genitalia and maintain dignity.)
Position: Lower bed flat, with patient resting on one pillow. Arms by sides.

Inspect
Distension, scars. drains and stomas (follow the drain and see what is draining and identify the type of stoma), masses, vessels, striae, hernias.
Ask the patient to raise their head off the pillow, breathe in and out, suck their tummy and give a cough. As they do this look for herniae and diversification of the herniae.

Palpation & Percussion
Assess for a triple A by placing hands either side of the umbilicus.
Feel for hernias in the inguinal region and ask patient to cough.
Squat by side of bed so patient's abdomen is at eye level.
Look at the patient's face and begin light palpation at the point farthest from pain. Palpate in four quadrants. Once your have palpated lightly repeat pressing more firmly.
If you suspect any herniae ask the patient to cough and follow the detailed hernia exam detailed later in the text.
Palpating a mass: feel for size, shape, surface, consistency, mobility, pulsatile nature, movement with respiration.

Liver: begin in the right iliac fossa, exert gentle pressure and ask the patient to breathe in and out. With inspiration drift your palm upwards towards the liver.
Percuss the liver – map out the upper and lower borders of liver by sequential plapation. Map out the top from the resonant lung field and then the bottom of liver from the right lower quadrant.
Normal: Around 5th IC midline to costal margin.

Spleen: begin in the right iliac fossa below the umbilicus. Ask the patient to breathe in and out moving towards the left costal margin.
Percuss the Spleen - percuss from the umbilicus to the left costal margin.

Kidneys: Place your left hand behind the right loin. Place your right hand at the costal margin. Push down with your right hand balloting the kidney. Repeat for the left kidney.

Percussion
Ascites – Percuss centrally, from the umbilicus to the flank on the left side. Ask the patient to roll towards you and percuss their back if ascites present.

Auscultate
Listen for 15-20 seconds for bowel sounds
Listen for renal bruits – press down firmly a few cm above the umbilicus at the lateral edge of the rectus muscle.
Listen for femoral bruits over the femoral pulse.

State to Examiners
That you would examine the external genitalia, dipstick the urine and perform a PR examination.

EXAMINATION

1.7 | Lump B

> ### Scenario
>
> A 56-year-old gentleman is referred to your general surgical clinic with a painful lump in his right groin.
>
> The patient is comfortable, you have washed you hands, introduced yourself and explained what you are going to do. Please examine this gentleman's groin.

Describe how you would begin

Expose and Inspect: Expose the patient from 'nipples to knees'. Dignity must be maintained and a chaperone used. Giving the patient a blanket/sheet to cover himself or herself prior to asking them to lower their underwear will help build trust and rapport. The patient can use this to cover themselves and only be exposed when necessary and for the shortest time possible.

Patient Standing: Ask the patient to stand and observe for any obvious swelling in the groin. You may also want to look around the bed for any hernia supports.

Look for previous herniae or abdominal scars. Note any laparoscopic hernia surgery scars found in the midline. Ask the patient to cough and observe for any swellings on both sides.

> 👓 **Inspection Findings**
>
>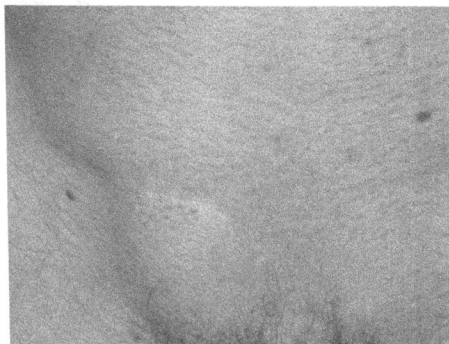

Describe the what you see on inspection

On standing the gentleman has an obvious swelling/lump in the right groin.

On inspection the swelling appears to be medial and superior to the pubic tubercle.

Overlying the lump in the groin crease there appears to be a scar suggesting a previous operation.

Having inspected what would you do next?

Palpate – ask whether the area is painful
If there is a palpable lump assess the lump for fluctuance, size, shape, mobility/tethering, whether it is reducible and whether you can get above it. It is good practice to ask the patient to first try and reduce the lump before you attempt this.

Try to ascertain where the lump originates from in comparison to the femoral pulse and whether it extends to the scrotum. It is a good idea to define your anatomy. Palpate the pubic tubercle at the medial aspect of the inguinal ligament and the anterior superior iliac spine (ASIS) demonstrating to the examiner you are considering where the lump appears in respect to the inguinal ligament.

Palpate both inguinal regions and compare both sides.

Ask the patient to cough while palpating the inguinal regions to check for a cough impulse.

Patient Supine
Once you have palpated the swelling with the patient stood up ask the patient to lie on the examination couch. Inspect and palpate both inguinal regions again and ask the patient to cough to test for a cough impulse.

Offer to examine the abdomen to look for signs of intraabdominal pressure that might predispose to a hernia.

Offer to examine the external genitalia.

> #### Findings
> The swelling is reducible both by yourself and the patient and when the patient is supine. There is a palpable cough impulse and, following reduction, pressure over the deep inguinal ring (mid-point of inguinal ligament – half-way between ASIS and pubic tubercle) does not maintain reduction following the patient coughing.
>
> You do not find any extension of the swelling into the scrotum and abdominal examination is unremarkable.

What is your differential diagnosis?

Use a surgical sieve and think of the potential structures that could be involved in this region:

- Skin – sebaceous cyst
- Subcutaneous – lipoma, fibroma
- Arterial – femoral pseudo/aneurysm
- Venous – saphena varix
- Lymphatic – lymphadenopathy
- Psoas abscess
- Hernia – inguinal, femoral
- Ectopic testis

Given the scar and examination findings this is likely to be a recurrent inguinal hernia. As reduction was not maintained with pressure over the deep ring it is likely to be a recurrent direct inguinal hernia.

How would you manage this patient?

Inguinal hernia repair can be open or laparoscopic. In this case the location of his scar suggests he has had previous open repair. He therefore should be consented for laparoscopic re-do surgery, as a general rule of thumb if his initial procedure had been laparoscopic the converse would be true[1].

Clinically how could you tell the difference between a femoral and an inguinal hernia?

Clinical distinction between inguinal and femoral hernias depends on the relationship to the pubic tubercle: inguinal hernias lie above and medial (emerging through the superficial ring), femoral hernias lie below and lateral (emerging from the cribriform fascia of the femoral sheath). In the acute setting this can be challenging and imaging may be used to confirm diagnosis.

Clinically how would you differentiate between a direct and an indirect inguinal hernia?

Knowledge of anatomy and surface markings is key. The below steps outline how to differentiate between direct and indirect herniae:
- Reduce the hernia and apply finger pressure over the deep inguinal ring (mid-point of inguinal ligament – half-way between ASIS and pubic tubercle)
- Ask the patient to cough
- Pressure over the deep ring should maintain reduction of indirect hernia (passes through deep ring) on coughing.
- Direct inguinal hernia will bulge out despite pressure over deep ring medial to point of pressure (passes through weakness in posterior wall of canal)

Although this question is an exam favorite in reality the sensitivity of this test is poor and the most reliable way to determine between the two is during the operation.

What is the definition of a hernia?

'The protrusion of a viscus or part of a viscus through a defect of the walls of its containing cavity into an abnormal position' [2]

If you were unsure of the diagnosis what investigation might you request?

An ultrasound scan of the groin is often used to confirm diagnosis, however computer tomography is increasingly utilised, especially in the acute setting[1][3]. Remember in the acutely unwell patient emergency surgery should not be delayed for further imaging if strangulation is clinically diagnosed.

What are the potential major complications of any hernia?

- Obstruction: Constriction at the neck of a hernia sac leads to obstruction of the loops of bowel within it.
- Strangulation: Constriction prevents venous return causing venous congestion, arterial occlusion and gangrene. This may lead to perforation and peritonitis.

What risks does a primary open inguinal hernia repair carry?

- Bleeding/haematoma
- Seroma formation which may require drainage
- Wound infection
- DVT/PE
- Complications related to the general anaesthetic (including the rare incidence of heart attack or death)

EXAMINATION

- Numbness can occur over the medial aspect of the wound and the groin, this may settle or be a permanent complication
- Chronic pain (inguinodynia). Pain is common post operatively but often subsides, if pain persists over 6 months it is classed as chronic. Severe or debilitating pain is thought to occur in 0.5-6% of patients, however some have found a degree of chronic pain in up to 54% of patietnts[1][4]. This pain can be difficult to control and should be managed in a chronic pain clinic. It is vital one consents the patient regarding this complication.
- Testicular atrophy: damage to the blood supply of the testicle resulting in a reduction in the size of the affected testicle. This risk is around 0.1%, or 1 in 1000 operations.
- Infection of the mesh: may require its removal risk is 0.5% risk with open surgery, 0.1% risk with laparoscopic surgery.
- Conversion to open surgery if laparoscopic
- Injury to other abdominal organs such as the colon or bladder present within the hernial sac.
- Recurrence of the hernia – about 2% risk at 5 years.

What are the boundaries of the inguinal canal?

Boundaries of inguinal canal (MALT):
Roof: internal oblique and transversus abdominis **M**uscle fibres
Anteriorly: external oblique **A**poneurosis and internal oblique
Floor: Inguinal **L**igament
Posteriorly: **T**ransversalis fascia

What are the contents of the inguinal canal?

Males: the spermatic cord and its coverings and the ilioinguinal nerve.
Females : the round ligament of the uterus and the ilioinguinal nerve.

What are the contents of the spermatic cord?

Spermatic Cord Contents.The classic description of the contents of spermatic cord in the male are:
- 3 arteries: artery to vas deferens (or ductus deferens), testicular artery, cremasteric artery.
- 3 fascial layers: external spermatic, cremasteric, and internal spermatic fascia.
- 3 other structures: pampiniform plexus, vas deferens (ductus deferens), testicular lymphatics.
- 3 nerves: genital branch of the genitofemoral nerve (L1/2), sympathetic and visceral afferent fibres, ilioinguinal nerve (N.B. outside spermatic cord but travels next to it)

From where does a Spigellian hernia emerge?

From the lateral part of the rectus sheath at the level of the arcuate line of Douglas

A Spigelian hernia (or lateral ventral hernia) is a hernia through the spigelian fascia, which is the aponeurotic layer between the rectus abdominis muscle medially, and the semilunar line laterally.
Spigelian hernias are usually small and therefore risk of strangulation is high. Most occur on the right side. (4th–7th decade of life).

SUMMARY OF EXAMINATION

Wash Your Hands
Ensure that you are seen by the examiners to wash your hands using alcohol gel provided.

Introduce, Explain, Expose and Inspect
Begin by introducing yourself, explain what you are going to do and check that this is ok with the patient and that he/she is not in any pain.
For herniae examination the patient should ideally be bare from 'nipples to knees'.

Patient Standing
Ask the patient to stand and observe for any obvious swelling in the groin.

Inspect
For previous hernia or abdominal scars. Ask the patient to cough and observe for any swellings.

Palpate
If there is a palpable lump assess the lump for fluctuance, size, shape, mobility/tethering, whether it is reducible and whether you can get above it. Also try to ascertain where the lump originates from in comparison to the femoral pulse and whether it extends to the scrotum.
Palpate both inguinal regions and compare both sides.
Ask the patient to cough while palpating the inguinal regions to check for a cough impulse.

Patient Supine
Ask the patient to lie on the examination couch.
Inspect and palpate both inguinal regions again and ask the patient to cough to again test for a cough impulse.
Offer to examine the abdomen to look for signs of intraabdominal pressure that might predispose to a hernia.
Offer to examine the external genitalia.

Closing
Thank the patient. Inform them that they may now get dressed or ensure they are adequately covered.
Present your findings to the examiner.

TOP TIPS

➕ Scars in the groin can be easy to miss as they are often in skin creases, look carefully over any lump

➕ Asking the patient to identify the 'area of concern' or reduce the lump themselves can help to quickly identify pathology

➕ Remember to examine the external genitalia and also abdomen to avoid missing an inguinoscrotal hernia or abdominal mass causing pressure

EXAMINATION

References

1. Burney R. Inguinal hernia. BMJ Best Practice 2015. http://bestpractice.bmj.com/best-practice/mybp/monograph-pdf/723.pdf (accessed 12/12/2015).
2. Longmore JM. *Oxford handbook of clinical medicine.* 8th ed. / Murray Longmore ... [et al.]. ed. Oxford: Oxford University Press, 2010.
3. Bradley M, Morgan D, Pentlow B, et al. The groin hernia - an ultrasound diagnosis? Ann R Coll Surg Engl 2003;**85**(3):178-80.
4. Poobalan AS, Bruce J, Smith WC, et al. A review of chronic pain after inguinal herniorrhaphy. The Clinical journal of pain 2003;**19**(1):48-54.

1.8 Hernia

Scenario

A 55-year-old female presents to the general surgical clinic complaining of a lump increasing in size at the site of a Kocher's incision that was performed for an open cholecystectomy 15 years ago. She has no obstructive symptoms.

You have washed your hands, introduced yourself and explained what you are going to do. Please exam this lady's abdominal lump.

Describe how you would begin

Expose and inspect: Ensure the patient is exposed from the nipple line to pubic symphysis, a chaperone should be present and only fully expose the patient when necessary to maintain their modesty and dignity; a blanket is often useful. Look around the bed space for items such as abdominal binders (although now rare). Remember to inspect the whole abdomen and not just the site of the mass.

Begin inspection with the patient standing and then ask them to cough at this point.

Next ask the patient to lie supine. Make a point of observing from the side to look for hernia swellings and ask them to cough again.

👓 Findings

The patient has increased body habitus and smells of cigarette smoke. She has a visible mass at the lateral aspect of her Kochers incision site. There are no visible skin changes. The swelling is more prominent on coughing. She is comfortable and not distended.

Describe you findings.

Concise communication of the key positives and poignant negatives will impress the examiner. This can be done at the end of the exam or following end of bed inspection.

Describe what you would do next.

Now focus your exam on the site of the swelling. If the lump is not prominent when supine examine the patient standing.

Palpate: Palpation aims to characterize the size, shape, mobility and consistency / fluctuancy of the lump. Ensure you palpate the whole length of the scar site, is there more than one site of scar defect? Palpation also can guide you to whether the swelling is tender or if there are significant physical characteristics, i.e. erythema or skin degradation/ changes. At this point one can also test for trans-illumination.

Cough: While placing a hand over the lump ask the patient to cough, is there a cough impulse?

Reducibility: This can be painful and one must not cause the patient avoidable pain. It is good practice to first ask the patient if they can reduce the hernia. If they cannot you must then attempt to reduce the hernia.

EXAMINATION

Percuss: Percuss both over the lump site and unaffected area of abdomen.

Auscultate: Auscultate both over the lump site and unaffected area of abdomen.

> ### Findings
>
> There is a reducible non-tender mass over the lateral aspect of the scar site. There is a palpable cough impulse. There are no skin changes. Bowel sounds are present over the mass. It does not trans-illuminate. There are no stigmata of obstruction.

How would you end the examination?

Thank the patient and cover them up, turn to the examiner and place your hands behind your back. State how you would like to complete your examination, this would include a full abdominal examination. Only offer to perform digital rectal examination (DRE) if it is relevant to the scenario and remember to state a chaperone must be present, in this case a DRE is not indicated.

Present your findings

Ensure this is concise and includes your positive findings and relevant negative findings.

What do you think is your primary diagnosis? What are your differential diagnoses?

In light of my examination findings and the location over a previous surgical scar this is likely to be an incisional hernia.

Other differentials for a superficial abdominal mass in this region include:

Skin: Cyst, insect bite
Subcutaneous: Lipoma, seroma, abscess, rectus sheathe haematoma
Neoplastic: Rectus sheathe sarcoma
Hernia: Incisional, spigelian
Vascular: Aneurysm

How would you manage this patient?

Ultrasonography (USS) is often used to confirm the presence of an incisional hernia1. Computer tomography (CT) allows more detailed visualization of the anatomy and characteristics that aids in management and pre-operative planning[1][2].

When there is no acute complications incisionalhernias' can be managed conservatively or surgically. The decision should be made in conjunction with the patient considering both the risks and benefits of available options.

Conservative measures aim to reduce factors which raise intra-abdominal pressure such as weight loss and treating chronic coughs. Smoking cessation is essential as it results in coughing and impairs collagen function[3]. Some use abdominal binders/corsetry.

Surgically there are many accepted ways to repair incisional hernia but they are best divided into laparoscopic versus open. Mesh has been shown to be vastly superior to suture repair, suture repair must only be considered if the hernia is small (<3cm) with some surgeons still using mesh[1][4][5]. If surgery is undertaken modifiable factors as mentioned in conservative management must also be addressed to minimize recurrence risk with concentration on weight reduction and smoking cessation. When surgery is considered it is key to involve the anaesthetic team as these patients often have considerable anaesthetic risk.

Can you give a definition of a hernia?

'The protrusion of a viscus or part of a viscus through a defect of the walls of its containing cavity into an abnormal position' [6]

9. What types of general surgical hernia do you know?

Examples of general surgical hernias include:

Hiatus (sliding and rolling)
Umbilical and para-umbilical
Inguinal (direct and indirect)
Femoral
Incisional
Spigelian
Richters'
Littres'

Hernias can be further classified as to whether they are reducible, incarcerated, strangulated or obstructive.

What are the risk factors for hernia formation?

Generalised risk factors for abdominal herniation include the following:

- Raised intra-abdominal pressure
  - Straining, chronic cough, obesity, ascites.
- Poor connective tissue tone/integrity
  - Poor nutrition, congenital soft tissue and cartilaginous disorders
- Smoking
  - This is a vital contributory factor as it affects both intra-abdominal pressures and soft tissue competency.

Incisional hernias have additional risk factors:

- Technical factors
  - High risk incision i.e. Subcostal
  - Poor closure technique
- Tissue factors
  - Increased age
  - Diabetes
  - Infection at site
  - Immunosuppression
- Post operative complications – which are higher if primary surgery was emergency surgery.
  - Sepsis
  - Malnutrition
- Inappropriate activity post procedure i.e. early return to heavy lifting.

What are the complications associated with hernias if they are not operated on?

Complications include:

EXAMINATION

Increasing size of hernia
Incarceration
Strangulation
Obstruction
Spontaneous or traumatic rupture of hernia/hernia sac (very rare).

Non-acutely the symptoms patients are most likely to complain of are pain or a lump.

What is the difference between incarceration and strangulation?

Incarceration is when the hernia is irreducible however there is not necessarily any complication from this. Conversely in strangulation the blood supply to the hernia is compromised resulting in ischemia, necrosis and perforation. Strangulation is a surgical emergency.

Can you name the following surgical incisions?

1) Mercedes Benz   2) Kochers   3) Rooftop (double Kochers)   4) Midline
5) Paramedian   6) Transverse   7) Gridiron (McBurneys)   8) Lanz
9) Pfannenstiel   10) Thoracoabdominal

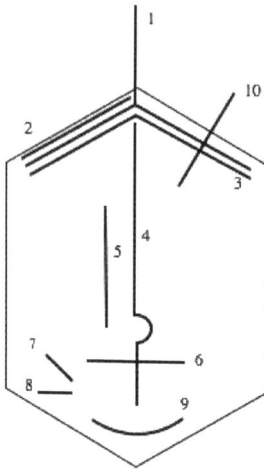

What types of wound healing do you know?

Healing by primary intention
• Wound edges opposed. Minimal scarring with optimum aesthetic outcome.
Healing by secondary intention
• Wound heals via granulation tissue, contraction and epithelization. Can lead to significant scarring affecting cosmesis.
Healing by tertiary intention
• Wound initially left open and then edges re-approximated when conditions favorable.

Can you tell me the difference between hypertrophic and keloid scarring?

Hypertrophic scarring is characterized by excessive scar tissue that remains in the boundaries of the original wound. Keloid scarring is where there is excessive scar tissue that extends beyond the original wound.

SUMMARY OF EXAMINATION

- Wash your hands and introduce yourself to the patient gaining consent for examination.
- Position, expose and inspect the patient from the end of the bed. Ask the patient to cough.
- Do this with the patient standing and then supine.
- Palpate assessing the characteristics of the abdominal lump/hernia. Palpate for a cough impulse.
- Assess if the hernia is reducible.
- Percuss.
- Auscultate.
- Thank the patient, cover them up, turn to the examiner and explain how you would like to complete your exam and give your findings.
- Top Tips
- When examining a hernia always initially examine with the patient standing.
- Ask the patient to reduce the hernia before you attempt reduction.
- Remember that abdominal scars can become discrete in time and can be hidden in skin creases.

EXAMINATION

TOP TIPS

➕ When examining a hernia always initially examine with the patient standing.

➕ Ask the patient to reduce the hernia before you attempt reduction.

➕ Remember that abdominal scars can become discrete in time and can be hidden in skin creases.

References
1. Sanders DL, Kingsnorth AN. The modern management of incisional hernias. BMJ 2012;**344**:e2843.
2. Aguirre DA, Santosa AC, Casola G, et al. Abdominal wall hernias: imaging features, complications, and diagnostic pitfalls at multi-detector row CT. Radiographics : a review publication of the Radiological Society of North America, Inc 2005;**25**(6):1501-20.
3. Franz MG. The biology of hernia formation. The Surgical clinics of North America 2008;**88**(1):1-15, vii.
4. Luijendijk RW, Hop WC, van den Tol MP, et al. A comparison of suture repair with mesh repair for incisional hernia. N Engl J Med 2000;**343**(6):392-8.
5. Schumpelick V, Klinge U, Rosch R, et al. Light weight meshes in incisional hernia repair. Journal of minimal access surgery 2006;**2**(3):117-23.

1.9 | Stoma

Scenario

You have come to review a postoperative patient's stoma on the ward. The patient had their procedure five days ago. The indication for stoma formation was secondary to inflammatory bowel disease; the operation went smoothly. The patient is comfortable, you have washed your hands, introduced yourself and explained what you are going to do. Please examine this patient's stoma site.

Describe how you would begin

Expose and position: Expose the patient from nipple to groin crease. Ask for a chaperone. Ensure a blanket is available for the patient for discretion when not being examined/inspected.. Only expose the patient when necessary. Lie the patient flat.. Ask the patient if it would be possible to remove the bag and check they have spare bags and the correct equipment to do so.

Inspect: Start by inspecting the patient from the end of the bed and then move directly on to a focused inspection of the abdomen and the stoma. When observing the stoma ask the patient to cough in an attempt to expose a para-stomal hernia.

Inspection

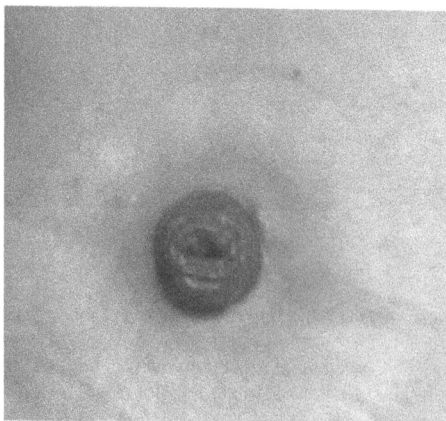

Describe what you can see on close inspection of the stoma.

There is a pink, healthy looking stoma. The stoma is spouted and appears to only have one lumen. The skin around the stoma site looks healthy.

EXAMINATION

Having inspected describe what you will do next.

Palpate around the stoma attempting to illicit tenderness or discover the presence of the parastomal hernia.

Percuss.

Auscultate for bowel sounds.

> ### ᏮᏗ Findings
>
> On palpation there is no tenderness or masses around the stoma and it is not prolapsed. Bowel sounds are normal and the stoma is functioning. You are happy that the stoma is healthy and progressing well.

What else would you offer to do?

Digital examination of the stoma. Remember this can be very tender and should be performed with a gloved little finger and lubricating jelly.
Full examination of the gastro-intestinal system.

What sort of stoma do you think is demonstrated in this case?

Due to its spouted appearance this is likely to be an ileostomy and is llikely ocated in the RIF

What would you say to the patient following a normal examination?

When examination is normal it is important to reassure the patient and state that everything appears normal, especially as this stoma has recently been formed the patient will be naturally concerned and it will take a while for them to know what is 'normal'. Give the patient an opportunity to ask questions. It is also advisable to briefly touch on common complications/difficulties some patients experience and ensure they have contact with the stoma nurses and know how to contact them if needed.

A vital topic to be discussed is the stoma output and consistency. Enquire as to whether they are using agents to slow transit such as loperamide/codeine or thickening aids such as marshmallows.

Can you give a definition of a stoma?

Stoma is derived from the Greek language and means a mouth like opening, the mouth and anus are naturally formed stomas. In the context of surgery a stoma describes the artificial opening of a tube that has been brought to the body surface[1].

What types of stoma do you know?

There are many types of stoma so it is important this answer is structured.

Anatomically the following are examples of surgically formed stomas':

Tracheostomy
Gastrostomy
Jejunostomy
Ileostomy

EXAMINATION

Caecostomy (rare)
Colostomy
Urostomy
Nephrostomy

These can then be further classified by function (i.e feeding) and by whether they are an end, looped or double-barreled stoma.

What indications in a general surgery setting for stoma formation can you think of?

Diversion
Exteriorisation
Feeding
Lavage
Decompression

Describe the key principle behind stoma site selection?

Selecting the optimal stoma site depends on many factors. The patient and stoma nurses should be involved in this process. The co-operation and input of the stoma nurse team is key in eliciting the optimal stoma site. Some factors to consider are as follows[2]:

Avoid existing scars, wounds and bony prominences
Avoid skinfolds/creases
Assess location while the patient is wearing clothes, i.e. avoid belt line
Ensure the patient can easily access the stoma site
Take into account patients occupation and factors such as amputations and wheel chair status
Consider the anatomy of the procedure undertaken

What clues on inspection can help you differentiate between an ileostomy and colostomy?

Colostomy	Ileostomy
Flush to skin	Spouted
Classically LIF	Classically RIF
Formed stool output	Liquid effluent
Large caliber	Small caliber

The above is only a guide and there is great variability. Perhaps the best way to deduce what sort of stoma you are looking at is to inspect the effluent. Note that ileal conduits will look like ileostomies but the effluent will be urine. However the only way to be 100% certain is to review the case notes.

EXAMINATION

What common complications do you know which can complicate ileostomies and colostomies?

Early Complications	Late Complications
Ischaemia and gangrene	Parastomal hernia
Bleeding	Prolapse
Infection	Retraction
Skin irritation	Stenosis
High output	High output and nutritional disorders
	Leakage and skin irritation
	Psychological and sexual difficulties

Why are ileostomies formed with a spout?

Ileostomy effluent is an irritant to the surrounding skin due to its volume, enzyme content and pH. Forming a spout when combined with a skin protector and correctly fitting bag aims to prevent the effluent coming into contact with the skin.

What is a urostomy?

This stoma is used for the diversion of the urinary system. Indications for their formation include obstructive tumours, trauma, incontinence which has not been managed with conservative means and refractory radiation cystitis[3].

Can you describe the principles of urostomy formation using an ileal conduit?

Pre-operatively the patient must be adequately counseled and consented. The stoma site must be assessed and marked.

Intra-operatively a segment of ileum is isolated along with its blood supply. Ileo-ileal anastomosis is performed to restore continuity of the intestine. The ureters are divided and the distal ends ligated. The proximal ends of the ureters are implanted into the proximal end of the isolated ileal segment. The distal end of the ileum is then brought through the pre-decided stoma site and everted to form the spout of the urostomy, this can appear similar to a ileostomy[4].

SUMMARY OF EXAMINATION

- Wash you hands and introduce yourself to the patient gaining consent for examination
- Position, expose and inspect the patient from the end of the bed
- Move on to closer inspection of the stoma and its effluent
  - Offer to examiner/patient to remove the bag if present as long as appropriate equipment and replacement bags are present.
- Palpate around the stoma
- Percuss and auscultate if indicated
- Offer to perform more invasive aspects of examination such as digital stoma examination if you feel it is indicated
- Thank the patient and cover them up, be prepared to help them replace their bag
- Turn to the examiner and explain how you would like to complete your exam and give your findings

EXAMINATION

EXAMINATION

TOP TIPS

➕ Listen carefully to what the examiner is asking you to do. If they ask you to examine a stoma this is a focused examination and thus one should not perform a full abdominal examination.

➕ State to the examiner that ideally you would see the patient as a dual appointment with the stoma nurse, this will help demonstrate you appreciate the importance of multi-disciplinary input which is vital in stoma management.

➕ When being examined on stomas' never forget the psychological stress having a stoma can cause the patient and always try to mention the crucial role of the stoma nurses in any long-term management questions.

➕ Ideally the bag should be removed for the examination, however in an exam setting this can be painful and embarrassing for the patient as they are examined repeatedly. Thus if there is a bag it is wise to ask the examiner if they would like you to remove the bag.

➕ Always thoroughly inspect for a double lumen stoma as these are easily missed under pressure, the efferent limb will reduce in size as it is not being used.

References
1. Martin EA. *Concise medical dictionary.* 7th ed. ed. Oxford: Oxford University Press, 2007.
2. Cataldo PA. Technical tips for stoma creation in the challenging patient. Clinics in colon and rectal surgery 2008;**21**(1):17-22.
3. Colwell JG, M. Carmel J. *Fecal & Urinary Diversions: Management Principles:* Elsevier Health Sciences, 2012.
4. Urinary Incontinence in Neurological Disease: Management of Lower Urinary Tract Dysfunction in Neurological Disease. London, 2012:252.

1.10 Anterior Triangle

Anterior Triangle Scenario

A 56 year old female attends the Head and Neck outpatients clinic. She reports a 2 month history of a painless, firm swelling in the anterior part of her lower neck.

The patient is comfortable, you have washed your hands, introduced yourself and explained what you are going to do. Please examine this ladies neck.

Describe how you would begin

Expose and inspect :
- Adequately expose the patient's head and neck along with the upper part of the chest.
- View the patient from the front and side commenting on any gross swelling along with any skin ulceration or pigmentation.

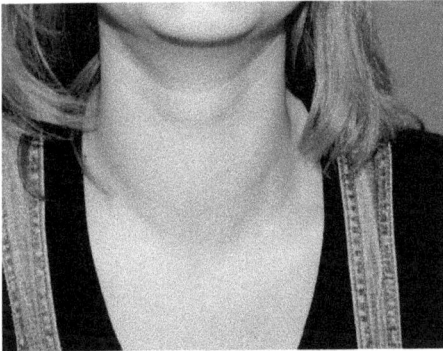

Describe what you see on inspection

There is a diffuse swelling on the lower aspect of the anterior triangle.

Having inspected, what would you do next?

Palpation:
- Begin by focusing the examination on the anterior triangle. Feel for any swelling and comment upon:

1. Firmness
2. Uninodular or multinodular
3. Fixity to skin
4. Fixity to underlying structures
5. Overlying ulceration
6. Pulsatility
7. Location – midline or laterally placed.
8. Pigmentation/homogenous/heterogenous/irregular margin

- Examine for any other swellings in the anterior triangle and say you would like to fully

EXAMINATION

examine the posterior triangles and perform a full examination of the head including the tonsillar bed.

EXAMINATION

Voice:
- Assess the patients voice by asking the patient to repeat a simple phrase such as '40 West Street'.

Percussion:
- Assess for any retrosternal extension by percussing upwards from the sternum.

Auscultation:
- Listen over the swelling for any evidence of fluid thrill or bruit.

Attachment to other structures:
- Assess for any attachment to the tongue by asking the patient to stick their tongue out and observing for any movement of the neck swelling.
- Assess for the relationship to the larynx by asking the patient to take a sip of water and then swallow it.
- Complete the examination by saying "I would like to carry out a full examination looking for peripheral stigmata of Thyroid disease".

> Findings
> 2.5cm hard uninodular swelling.
> Right lower anterior triangle.
> No fixity to the overlying skin. No pigmentation or ulceration.
> Moves with swallowing.
> No movement with tongue protrusion.
> Fine tremor
> Atrial Fibrillation at rate 95

What is your differential diagnosis?
- **Skin and subcutaneous tissue** – Melanoma, Sebaceous cyst, Lipoma
- **Thyroid** – Goitre, Nodule, Carcinoma
- Thyroglossal Cyst
- **Lymph Node** – Lower end of Deep Cervical Chain. Malignant inflitration, Lymphoma
- **Vascular** – Chemodectoma

- The duration of symptoms, size and features of hyperthyroidism, suggest this is likely to be a uninodular toxic thyroid nodule.

As part of your work up, you order Thyroid Function Tests. These reveal a low TSH with a high free T4 and T3 confirming a Hyperthyroid state. Can you describe the mechanism of production of T3 and T4 through the release of TSH?
- Iodide trapping from the bloodstream
- Oxidation of I- to I2
- Secretion of I2 into colloid
- Binding of I2 to Tyrosine to form Mono-iodotyrosine(MIT) or Di-iodotyrosine (DIT) forming thyroglobulin
- TrH released from Hypothalamus
- TSH (glycoprotein hormone) released from Anterior Pituitary

- TSH binds to surface receptors causing Pinocytosis of Thyroglobulin
- Proteolysis of thyroglobulin by Lysosyme causes release of MIT and DIT
- Combination of 2 DIT molecules to form T4 along with 1 molecule of MIT and DIT to form T3
- T3 and T4 released into bloodstream bound to Thyroid Binding Globulin (TBG), Thyroid Binding Pre Albumin (TBPA) and Albumin.

What further Investigations would you like to use to further assess this swelling?

I would like to assess this swelling with the use of

- Blood tests including FBC, U+E, LFT, Calcium
- Ultrasound.
- FNA biopsy under ultrasound guidance.
- CT of neck, thorax and abdomen if suspicion of malignant disease.

How will you manage the patient?

Medical
- Atrial fibrillation can be managed with anticoagulation. If the patient has no evidence of high output heart failure you may wish to add a low dose Beta Blocker to achieve a heart rate of 60-80 .Carbimazole can be used if the patient becomes more thyrotoxic prior to Surgical intervention.

Surgical
- If confirmed as unilateral then request a thyroid lobectomy of the affected side.

> Anterior triangle
> Medial border – Midline
> Lateral border – Anterior margin of Sternocleidomastoid
> Superior border – Lower border of Mandible.
>
> Subdivisions
> Muscular triangle
> Carotid triangle
> Submental triangle
> Submandibular triangle.

List the boundaries of the Anterior triangle. How might this be further subdivide

The pathology report notes the presence of severe dysplasia with invasion of the basement membrane of the Thyrocytes. Following CT imaging and discussion with the patient, you take informed consent for a Total Thyroidectomy.

What General and Specific complications to the operation will you consent the patient for?

General
- Pain, swelling, sutures
- DVT/PE
- Infection
Specific

EXAMINATION

- Hoarse voice
- Difficulty with achieving high pitched notes (for groups like professional singers)
- Bleeding/haematoma and potential return to theatre.

How would you distinguish between the different types of malignant disease of the thyroid?

- Papillary Carcinoma – Around 70% of malignancies. Tends to affect younger patients. Multifocal lesions with pale 'Orphan Annie' nuclei. Psammoma calcification is diagnostic. TSH dependent.
- Follicular Carcinoma – Around 20% of malignancies. Mostly unifocal lesions. Follicular adenomas are extremely similar to carcinomas. FNA biopsy is of limited use because you are unable to distinguish if the lesion is benign or malignant..
- Medullary Carcinoma – 5% of malignancies. Multifocal lesions. Derived from parafollicular cells and consequently secrete Calcitonin. Can be part of MEN syndrome. Treated by total thyroidectomy. Monitor post operatively with Calcitonin levels. T4 is given post op as a replacement rather than for TSH suppression.
- Anaplastic Carcinoma – <5% of malignancies. Tends to affect older patients. Metastesises directly and to the lymphatics. Poor prognosis. Treatment focused on debulking and palliative radiotherapy. Occasionally may require tracheal stenting.

What important structures lie in close proximity and risk being damaged from a total thyroidectomy.

- Recurrent laryngeal nerve
- External laryngeal nerve
- Parathyroid Glands

Outline the course of the recurrent laryngeal nerve on both sides. Can you explain the embryological reasons for this relationship?

- Left side – loops under the arch of the aorta before running back up into the neck via the tracheo-oesophageal groove
- Right side – loops under the right subclavian artery before running back up into the neck via the tracheo-oesophageal groove

The recurrent laryngeal nerve is the nerve of the sixth pharyngeal arch whereas the arch of the aorta is derived from the left side of the 4th pharyngeal arch along with the right subclavian artery on the right side of the 4th arch. As these 2 structures descend into the neck they drag the recurrent laryngeal nerve downwards with them.

The recurrent laryngeal nerve is the nerve of the sixth pharyngeal arch. The primitive RLN enters the 6th arch on each side below the 6th aortic arch artery. On the left side, the arch artery retains its position as the ductus arteriosus so the nerve is found below the aortic arch after birth. On the right side, the 6th and 5th arch artery disappear. Leaving the RLN on the right to lie below the 4th arch artery which becomes the subclavian artery.

What hormone and electrolyte should be measured post operatively? Why might these be low ? What are the systemic consequences of a low level of this hormone.

- Measure parathyoid hormone and calcium – f
- Inadvertent excision of all of the 3 to 5 parathyroid glands.
- Hypocalcaemia – can lead to perioral and extremity tingling, cramps, tetany, carpopedal spasm, convulsions, long QT on ECG.

What signs might you identify with a low level of this hormone?

- Chvosteks sign – twitching of the muscles of facial expression when the facial nerve is tapped over its root.
- Trousseaus sign – spasm of the wrist and digits when a sphygmomanometer is applied to the same limb.

The pathology of the specimen returns as being a low grade follicular carcinoma. What further treatment should be given and how should the patient be followed up?

- Medical treatment – Thyroxine for TSH suppression along with replacement.
- Radiotherapy
- Clinic reviews

SUMMARY OF EXAMINATION

Site of lump
- Midline, supraclavicular
- Size
- Skin changes
- Scars

Protrusion of the tongue
- Ask patient to open mouth and stick tongue out as far as possible
- Moves on protrusion = thyroglossal cyst
- Does not move on protrusion = thyroid lump

Swallowing
- Place glass of water in patient's hands
- Ask to take sip of water, hold in mouth, swallow
- If moves on swallowing = thyroid gland issue / thyroglossal cyst

Palpate
1. From the back
- Be gentle, watch for discomfort
- Use fingertips (obviously!) to elicit physical signs
- Demonstrate the boundaries of the triangles of the neck

2. Palpate the triangles
- Anterior triangle: anterior border of Sternocleidomastoid, midline, ramus of mandible
- Posterior triangle: anterior border of trapezius, clavicle, posterior border of sternocleidomastoid

3. Determine whether the lump is solid or cystic
4. Confirm your findings (if necessary) by examining from the front

Auscultation
1. Thyroid bruit (Grave's thyroiditis)
2. Carotid bruit (carotid stenosis)

Differential diagnosis of neck lumps in anterior triangle:
Lymph nodes
Lipoma – painless / smooth mass
Sebaceous cyst
Salivary gland swelling – doesn't move on swallowing
Branchial cyst – present from birth – noticed in early adulthood
Carotid aneurysm – pulsatile mass – bruit present on auscultation
Carotid body tumour – transmits pulsation – can be moved side to side but not vertically
Laryngocele – reducible tense mass – mass returns on sneezing or nose blowing

EXAMINATION

1.11 | Neck Lump A

Parotid Swelling Scenario

A 72 year old Female attends the Maxillofacial clinic, she is concerned about an increasing swelling of her right pre-auricular area.

The patient is comfortable, you have washed your hands, introduced yourself and explained what you are going to do. Please examine this ladies neck.

Describe how you would begin

- Adequately expose the patients head and neck
- View the patient from the front and side commenting on any gross swelling along with any skin ulceration or pigmentation.

Describe what you see on inspection.

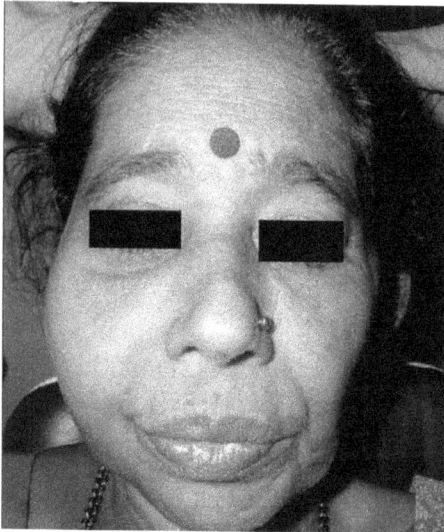

Having inspected, what would you do next?

Palpation: Focus the examination upon the patient's normal side explaining to the patient that you will then progress to the side of the abnormality. Examine the right pre-auricular region feeling for any gross swelling commenting upon:

EXAMINATION

1. Firmness
2. Size
3. Fixity to skin
4. Fixity to underlying structures
5. Overlying ulceration
6. Location - pre/post auricular or tail of Parotid
7. Pigmentation/homogenous/heterogenous/irregular margin

Examine the head and neck for any lymphadenopathy.

TOP TIP

Always start by stating that you would like to examine the normal side first. If you are doing this, explain also to the patient *(so that they don't tell you that you're examining the wrong side!)*

EXAMINATION

What other structures would you examine as part of your overall assessment?

- The opening of the parotid duct
- The external ear, the external auditory canal and tympanic membrane
- The facial nerve
- Skin of face

Where would you find the opening of the Parotid Duct?

- Opposite the upper second molar tooth on the buccal mucosa

Describe the branches of the Facial Nerve and how you would examine for them?

- Temporal Branch – Ask patient to raise eyebrows.
- Zygomatic Branch – Ask patient to screw up eyes.
- Buccal Branch – Ask patient to puff out cheeks.
- Marginal Mandibular Branch – Ask patient to show their teeth
- Cervical Branch – Ask patient to show their teeth.

Following a thorough assessment and Ultrasound scan, you localise a poorly defined 3cm swelling to the superficial lobe of the right parotid gland. There is no evidence of any visible stone at the orifice of the parotid duct and no deficit in facial nerve function. The patient reports no hearing loss or tinnitus. What further investigations would you use to further classify this swelling?

- US guided FNA
- CT Head and Neck
- Possible MRI Head and Neck

The results of further investigations reveal a diffuse involvement of the superficial lobe with finger like projections extending into the

deep lobe. Outline the most likely pathology and list a differential diagnosis.

- Pleomorphic Salivary Adenoma – most likely diagnosis
- Warthin tumour – associated with smoking. Often bilateral and multifocal.
- Mucoepidermoid Carcinoma

How would you manage this swelling?

Dependent on FNA.
- If malignant – discussion at MDT with possibility of excision after confirmation and staging
- If benign, offer of excision.

As part of the consent process, you mention the possible systemic complications that are common to all surgical procedures. The patient also enquires as to the specific complications of having a total parotidectomy. What are these?

- Facial nerve palsy – temporary or permanent, partial or complete
- Frey's syndrome (Auriculotemporal syndrome)

Can you explain the mechanism behind Frey's syndrome?

Aberrant regeneration of parasympathetic nerve fibres along the auriculotemporal nerve leads to the phenomenon of gustatory sweating.

During the procedure, you encounter 2 vessels within the deep lobe of the parotid gland. What are these vessels and can you name the terminal branches of this specific artery?

- Retromandibular vein
- External carotid artery – terminal branches include the maxillary artery and superficial temporal artery.

3 months post procedure, the patient mentions that she is experiencing a dry mouth. On further questioning, she also notes that she has had 2 episodes of conjunctivitis over the same period and is using eye drops. What autoimmune condition do you suspect and what autoantibodies do you request on taking a blood sample?

- Sjogrens syndrome
- Anti – La, anti – Ro, RF, ANA

Can you explain the mechanism behind this autoimmune condition?

- Autoimmune chronic focal lymphocytic infiltration of exocrine glands with a predilection for salivary and lacrimal glands

How would you further sub classify Sjogrens syndrome? What other features of autoimmune disease might you look for?

- Primary – the condition arises alone
- Secondary – to other autoimmune conditions such as rheumatoid arthritis, SLE, polymyositis or, systemic sclerosis

1.12 | Neck Lump B

Submandibular Swelling Scenario

A 35 year old Male attends the ENT clinic. He has noticed an intermittent swelling over the last 2 years below the left side of his mandible.

The patient is comfortable, you have washed your hands, introduced yourself and explained what you are going to do. Please examine this gentleman's neck.

Describe how you would begin

Expose and inspect

- Expose the patients head and neck. Observe the swelling from the front, side and back noting any gross swelling, skin changes or pulsatility. Note the presence of any other swellings.

Describe what you see on inspection.

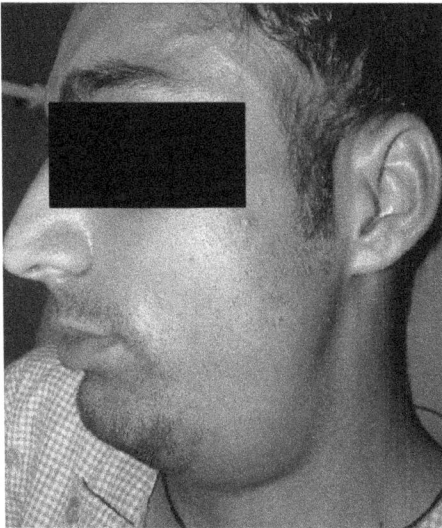

Having inspected, what would you do next?

Palpation

- Focus the examination on the patient's normal side explaining to the patient that you will then progress to the side of the abnormality. Examine the left submandibular region feeling for any gross swelling commenting upon:

EXAMINATION

- Firmness
- Size
- Fixity to skin
- Fixity to underlying structures
- Overlying ulceration
- Pigmentation/homogenous/heterogenous/irregular margin

- Tell the patient you would like to examine the rest of the head and neck for any other swelling or lymphadenopathy.

What other structures would you examine as part of your overall assessment?

- The opening of the submandibular duct
- The oral mucous membranes for any lesions
- The tonsillar fossae

Where would you find the opening of the submandibular duct?

Opposite the lower incisors on the lingual surface on the anterior aspect of the submandibular fold.

Findings
The swelling is a firm 5cm swelling over the left submandibular triangle. There is no pulsatility or skin changes. It is not fixed to the skin and intraorally a further hard swelling may be felt in the region of the posterior part of the submandibular duct. There is no discharge from the opening of the submandibular duct.

What is your differential diagnosis?

- Sialolithiasis
- Salivary gland tumour
- Dental abscess
- Lymphadenopathy
- Mucocele (Ranula)

TOP TIP

➕ Use a surgical sieve and think of the potential structures that could be involved in this region:

What initial investigations might you consider to provide more information regarding the swelling?

- Orthopantamogram (OPG) X-ray – to image a posterior floor of the mouth stone or, dental abscess
- Lower occlusal X-ray – to image an anterior floor of mouth stone.
- Ultrasound
- Sialogram – to image any filling defect of the submandibular gland – dependent upon the result of ultrasound

EXAMINATION

Further imaging reveals a 2cm stone in the posterior part of the duct with marked fibrosis of the submandibular acini. The patient is keen to have the gland removed. What specific complications to this procedure should you consent him for?

- Post operative decreased salivary flow/dry mouth
- Potential post operative weakness of the lower lip on the left side
- Weakness of the tongue and deviation of the tongue to the left side.
- Numbness of the tongue on that side.

What structures may be damaged that leads to these specific complications?

- Marginal Mandibular Branch of the Facial Nerve – weakened lower lip
- Hypoglossal Nerve – deviation of tongue to that side
- Lingual Nerve – loss of sensation of anterior 2/3 of tongue on that side.

The submandibular gland is divided into a superficial lobe and a deep lobe by which structure?

- Mylohyoid muscle

What are the borders of the submandibular triangle?

- Inferior edge of lower border of mandible
- Posterior belly of digastric
- Anterior belly of digastric.

What is the autonomic supply to the submandibular gland?

- Parasympathetic – via preganglionic fibres running in the Chorda Tympani branch of the facial nerve hitchhiking along the lingual nerve. Fibres synapse in the submandibular ganglion.
- Sympathetic –

During the operation, you come across 2 arteries that are branches of the external carotid artery. Can you name these branches?

- Facial artery
- Lingual artery

List the other branches of the External Carotid Artery in order from the Carotid Bifurcation.

- Ascending pharyngeal
- Occipital
- Posterior auricular
- Superior thyroid
- Lingual
- Facial
- Maxillary
- Transverse facial (occasionally)
- Superficial temporal.

At what C-Spine level does the Carotid Artery Bifurcate?

- C3 – C4

EXAMINATION

1.13 | Posterior Triangle

Posterior Triangle Swelling Scenario

A 68 year old male attends the maxillofacial outpatient department. He has noticed an increasing swelling on his right lower neck. He notes that this has been present for around 6 months. He is a known smoker of 50 pack years and has a heavy alcohol consumption of 35 units/week

The patient is comfortable, you have washed your hands, introduced yourself and explained what you are going to do. Please examine this gentlemans neck.

Describe how you would begin

Expose and inspect
* Expose the patient's head and neck. Observe the swelling from the front, side and back noting any gross swelling, skin changes or pulsatility. Note the presence of any other swellings.

Describe what you see on inspection.

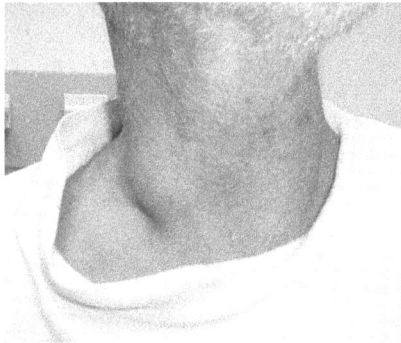

Having inspected, what would you do next?

Palpation
* Focus the examination on the patient's normal side explaining to the patient that you will then progress to the abnormal side. Examine the right posterior triangle feeling for any gross swelling commenting on:

> * Firmness
> * Size
> * Fixity to skin
> * Fixity to underlying structures
> * Ulceration of skin
> * Pigmentation of skin/homogenous/heterogenous/irregular margin

* Ask the patient if you can examine the rest of the head and neck for any other swelling,

lesion or, lymphadenopathy.

What other questions would you like to ask the patient as you are examining him?

- Any recent unintentional weight loss?
- Any difficulty swallowing?
- Any Hoarseness?
- Any night sweats or fever?
- Any numbness or paraesthesia in the arms?

What is your differential diagnosis of a swelling in the posterior triangle of the neck?

- Lymph node metastasis
- Lymphadenopathy of supraclavicular lymph nodes
- Lymphoma
- Tuberculosis
- Pharyngeal pouch
- Subclavian artery aneurysm
- Lipoma
- Cervical rib
- Cystic hygroma (in young infants)

TOP TIP

➕ Think logically with the most likely pathology at the top of your list. An alternative way to approach this in the exam is to think of the tissue types as you pass through skin, subcutaneous tissue, muscle, lymphatics, vessels and bone. Similar to the approach for a lump in the groin!

The patient has noticed a 'lump' at the back of his mouth on the right side. This has caused him to have some problems with eating hard foods and he feels like he is getting food stuck. What further investigations would you like to undertake in this gentleman?

- Imaging with a CT of the head, neck, thorax and upper abdomen
- A thorough examination of the Oropharynx via an Examination Under Anaesthetic (EUA)
- A biopsy of the lesion

Once this information has returned you see the patient back in the Head and Neck clinic. The results of the investigations reveal a poorly differentiated 3.5cm squamous cell carcinoma of the right tongue base extending across the midline with involvement of lymph nodes to level 5 on the right and no thoracic metastasis. What grading system could be used to further classify this lesion?

- TNM system

8. He mentions to you that he has had some difficulty with lifting his right shoulder tip upwards over the last 2 weeks. What nerve could be affected and what muscles does this supply?

- Spinal Root of the Accessory Nerve (CN XI)
- Sternocleidomastoid
- Trapezius

What are the borders of the posterior triangle

- Anteriorly – posterior border of sternocleidomastoid
- Inferiorly – superior border of the clavicle
- Posteriorly – Anterior border of trapezius

What are the names of the triangles that the posterior triangle is subdivided into and which structure subdivides them?

- Supraclavicular triangle
- Occipital triangle
- Divided by Inferior belly of Omohyoid

The level 5 lymph node lies in close proximity to the subclavian artery. The subclavian artery becomes the axillary artery at which anatomical landmark?

- The neck of the first rib.

The subclavian artery is further subdivided into 3 parts by a specific structure. What structure is this? What are the branches of each part?

- Scalenus anterior
- First part – vertebral Artery, thyrocervical trunk, Iinternal thoracic artery
- second part – costocervical trunk
- third Part – no branches

While resecting the tumour from the tongue base and performing a bilateral lymph node dissection, you can see the contents of the Carotid sheath. Following the internal jugular vein down, you come across a structure entering the junction between the left internal jugular vein and the left subclavian vein. What structure is this?

- thoracic duct

Unfortunately, during the operation, a small tear is made in this structure which continues to leak post operatively. What complication is this and how would you manage this?

- Chyle leak
- Manage with a medium chain triglyceride diet and a post-operative drain. Inspect the drain contents daily and measure volume.

You order an erect PA chest x-ray as part of your investigation into the chyle leak. On the chest x ray, you see that the left hemi-

diaphragm is elevated. What nerve may have been affected during the neck dissection and what nerve roots does this nerve contain?

- Phrenic nerve
- C3, C4 and C5

> **TOP TIP**
>
> ✚ '3,4 and 5 keep the Diaphragm alive'

EXAMINATION

1.14 | Ear Discharge

Ear Examination Scenario

A 42 year old female presents to her GP practice with a history of worsening hearing loss in her right ear over the last year. She reports an occasional yellowish discharge from her right ear.

The patient is comfortable, you have washed your hands, introduced yourself and explained what you are going to do. Please examine this ladies neck.

Describe how you would begin

Expose and inspect
- Examine both the patients external ears beginning with the normal/unaffected side. Tell the patient you will examine the abnormal side after the normal.
- Inspect the ear for any gross abnormality/sign of erythema or swelling of both the pinnae along with the mastoid processes.

Describe what you see on inspection.

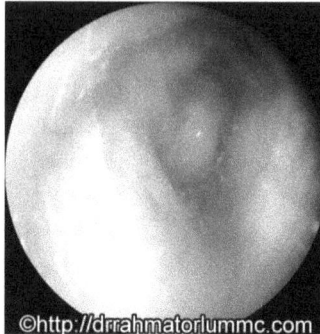

©http://drrahmatorlummc.com

Image taken from drahmatorlummc.com. ? require non copyright version

Having inspected, what would you do next?

Palpation
- Examine the external auditory canal and tympanic membrane with the use of an otoscope

You decide that you would like to utilise Webers and Rinnes tests to give further information on the nature of the hearing loss. How would you perform each of these and what information would they give?

- Webers Test – A 512 Hz tuning fork is vibrated and held in the middle of the patient's forehead. If the sound is heard louder in one ear, it suggests that there is either an ipsilateral Conductive hearing loss OR a contralateral Sensorineural hearing loss.

EXAMINATION

- **Rinnes Test** – A 512 Hz tuning fork base is vibrated and held against the mastoid process. After the patient notes that they can no longer hear the vibration, the other end of the tuning fork is held around an inch from the opening of the external canal. At this stage, they are then asked which noise was louder. A louder noise over the Mastoid process indicates an ipsilateral Conductive hearing loss.

Through the use of Webers and Rinnes tests, you believe that the patient has a conductive hearing loss in the right ear. With the use of the otoscope, you are able to visualise the tympanic membrane TM. What differentials might be contributing to the patient's hearing loss?

- Chronic Suppurative Otitis Media
- Cholesteatoma
- Otosclerosis

TOP TIP

Impacted ear wax is often the cause of conductive hearing loss. However, in this scenario the TM is visible and there is no impacted wax or debris in the external canal.

EXAMINATION

6. From the diagram, outline the anatomical features of the tympanic membrane. How might the differentials appear when viewed with an otoscope?

- Pars Tensa
- Pars Flaccida
- Umbo
- Cone of light
- Annulus

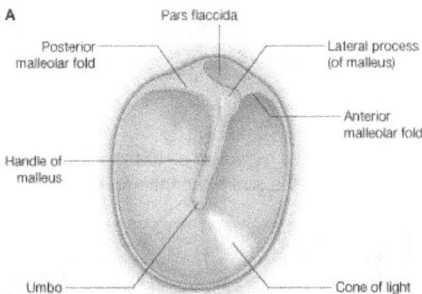

© Elsevier. Drake et al: Gray's Anatomy for Students - www.studentconsult.com

Diagram taken from Grays Anatomy – ? require non copyright version

- Chronic Suppurative Otitis Media – may have a kidney shaped perforation in the

pars yensa. The ear may discharge with an upper respiratory tract infection or, during swimming.
- Cholesteatoma – Perforation of the postero-superior part of the pars tensa or a small area in the pars flaccida. Leads to a foul smelling discharge.
- Otosclerosis – The tympanic membrane appears normal.

What is the pathogenesis of these conditions?

- Chronic Suppurative Otitis Media – Usually follows an episode of Acute Otitis Media (AOM) leading to a perforated tympanic membrane. Infection from pseudomonas, staphylococcus and proteus are common organisms. Irritation and inflammation may lead to further mucosal oedema and ulceration which can lead to the formation of granulation tissue and further irritation. A cycle of damage may then be formed.

- Cholesteatoma – Can be congenital or acquired. Acquired is more common – occurs secondary to an accumulation of keratin in a pouch of the tympanic membrane. This may then extend into the middle ear cavity. Congenital cholesteatomas occur secondary to the formation of keratin filled cysts.

- Otosclerosis – Fixation of the stapes in the oval window. Secondary to a familial condition where ankylosis occurs between the footplate and the oval window leading to conductive deafness.

You ascertain that there is a pearly white swelling on the superior aspect of the tympanic membrane. You suspect the diagnosis is that of a cholesteatoma. What complications might arise from this lesion?

- Erosion of the ossicles
- Damage to the facial nerve
- Invasion of the inner ear with potential spread intracranially leading to intracranial infection or venous sinus thrombosis.

The patient notes that she has had a loss of taste over the last few months. What specific nerve branch may be affected?

- Chorda tympani branch of the facial nerve.

What other nerve does this nerve branch hitchhike along? What other fibres other than taste fibres does it carry and where do they synapse?

- Lingual nerve (branch of the trigeminal nerve V3)
- Carries preganglionic parasympathetic nerve fibres to the submandibular and sublingual glands, which synapse in the submandibular ganglion.

TOP TIP

This is a detailed answer and may be beyond what is expected. To be aware that the chorda tympani carries parasympathetic fibres is probably adequate. The other cranial nerves that carry parasympathetic fibres are III, IX and X.

On formal audiometry, you establish that there is also a sensorineural element to her hearing loss in the contralateral ear. What may cause her sensorineural hearing loss?

- Noise injury/acoustic trauma
- Presbyacusis
- Ototoxic agents - aminoglycosides, frusemide, quinine, aspirin
- Menieres disease
- Acoustic neuroma

12. What nerves run through the internal auditory canal and where do they join the brainstem?

- Vestibulocochlear nerve
- Facial nerve
- Cerebellopontine angle

How would you classify a facial nerve Lesion. Can you differentiate between the two and name examples of potential causes of each type of lesion?

- Upper motor nerve lesion – forehead sparing as forehead receives bilateral innervation – example would be a cerebrovascular event
- Lower motor nerve lesion – forehead is affected as fibres have already crossed – examples would involve acoustic neuroma, bells palsy, cholesteatoma, skull base fracture, Ramsay Hunt syndrome or parotid mass/surgery.

The patient informs you that they have occasionally had a vesicular rash on one side of their forehead and that they previously have had an inability to move their facial muscles on that side at a separate time. What facial nerve lesion would lead to this temporary phenomenon? What virus could cause it?

- Bells Palsy
- Reactivation of herpes zoster

How would you manage this condition when it occurred?

- Reassure the patient that it is likely to be a temporary condition. Explain what the condition is.
- Eye cover and eye drops for the period of inability to blink – to prevent drying out of the cornea
- Short course of oral steroid (Prednisolone)

EXAMINATION

TOP TIP

Again, these are difficult questions. Knowing the difference between an upper and lower facial nerve lesion and how they effect the forehead is probably adequate.

1.15 | Spine

Scenario

A 25 year old lady is referred to your spinal clinic with low back pain which came on gradually during the last few months. The pain got worse in the last few days and the patient describes the pain as burning in nature, radiating to the right leg with difficulty in walking.

The patient is comfortable, you have washed your hands, introduced yourself and explained what you are going to do. Please examine this lady's back.

Describe how you would begin

Expose and Inspect: For a back examination the patient should be exposed to underwear.
Ask the patient to walk away a few steps, turn around and come back.

With the patient standing, look (from the front, back and sides) for the following:
any obvious deformity (e.g. scoliosis, kyphosis), swellings, scars, abnormal pigmentation like café au lait spots and muscle wasting.

ᏱᏜ Inspection Findings

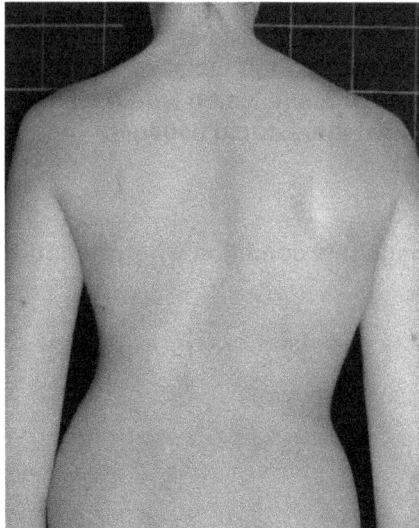

Describe the what you see on inspection

On standing this lady has an obvious thoracolumbar scoliosis with the convex side of the curve directed toward the left side. There is no obvious swelling, scar or muscle wasting.

Having inspected what would you do next?

Next steps are feel, move and specific tests.

A. Feel (palpation): By palpation you are looking for the following (ask about pain before you palpate):

Tenderness: Look for both bony and paraspinal muscle tenderness. Start from the cervical spine downward to the sacroiliac joint.

Stepping: Palpate between the spines of the vertebrae, slide your fingers down the spine and look for any abnormal spinous process step.

B. Move:

In standing position:
1. Forward flexion is tested by asking the patient to lean forward as far as the patient can and measure the distance from the fingertips to the floor. Normal value is about 7 cm. If the flexion is limited then mark the spine to determine whether the limitation is in the thoracic or lumbar spine (Schober's test, will be discussed later).

2. Extension is tested by asking the patient to bend backward. Normal range is about 30°.

3. Lateral flexion is testing by asking the patient to slide their hand down the side of their leg. Normal range is about 30°.

In sitting position:
Lateral rotation is testing by asking the patient to sit down, arm on each hip, the patient twists their shoulder as far round as they can, both to the left and to the right. Rotation is normally 40°.

C. Specific tests:

Supine position:
Straight leg raising test: This test assesses nerve root compression (L4-S1). It is performed by lifting the patient's leg while keeping the knee straight and stopping when the patient feels pain in the back/leg, then passively dorsiflex the foot which will worsen the pain. By maintaining the angle of dorsiflexion, flex the knee until the pain is relieved (Laségue's test).
Contralateral straight leg raising test: Pain in the affected buttock/leg when the opposite leg is raised. This test is the most specific test for herniated disc disorders.

Prone position:
Reverse Laségue's test: This test assesses nerve root compression (L2, L3). It is performed by flexing each knee in turn, ask if it causes pain in the anterior thigh.

Finally, to complete the examination: do a full neurological examination of the legs, check the femoral pulses and do an abdominal examination.

Mention the contribution of the thoracic and lumbar spine to the spine movements and what is Schrober's method?

Flexion: by doing Schrober's method: mark a point midline between the dimples of Venus and another point 10 cm above it. This approximates to the lumbar spine. Measure the distance between the two points in standing and when the spine is maximally flexed forwards. The increase should be 8-10 cm (< 3 cm suggests severe restriction). Do the same for the thoracic spine, marking the prominent T1 spinous process and a point 20 cm distal to that. The increase should be about 8 cm.

Extension: 25 degrees thoracic, 35 degrees lumbar.

Lateral flexion: the contributions of the thoracic and lumbar are about equal.

Rotation: is almost entirely thoracic.

How can you differentiate clinically between L5 and S1 nerve root compression?

L5 root is evaluated by testing the following:
Motor: Ankle dorsiflexion, foot inversion, toe extension.
Sensation: Lateral leg and dorsal foot.
Reflex: none

S1 root is evaluated by testing the following:
Motor: Foot plantar flexion and eversion.
Sensation: posterior leg and plantar foot.
Reflex: Achilles reflex.

> ### ⌒ Findings
>
> The patient has an obliterated lumbar lordosis, thoracolumbar scoliosis, limitation of mainly forward flexion. She has a positive straight leg raise test of the right leg, diminished right ankle jerk, weak plantar flexion and diminished sensation on the lateral border of the right foot

What is your differential diagnosis?

Possible causes of back pain with sciatica are:
1. Lumbar disc herniation which is the most likely cause in this scenario.
2. Spinal stenosis
3. Spondylolisthesis
4. Tumour (primary, secondary).
5. Spondyloarthropathy
6. Infection

Given the history and examination findings, this is likely to be a lumbar disc herniation L5/S1 with compression on the S1 nerve root. The ankle jerk, plantar flexion and the sensation on the lateral border of the foot innervated by S1.

How would you manage this patient?

I would like to confirm my diagnosis by proceeding with investigations as follow:
Plain radiography:
Indicated before proceeding with other special tests to rule out other disorders, such as isthmic disorders. However, most plain radiographic findings are nonspecific and plain radiography can usually be deferred for 6 weeks.
CT and myelography:
Helpful for identifying lateral pathologic conditions like lateral foraminal stenosis.
MRI:
It is the investigation of choice. It is superior for identifying cord disorders, neural tumours, and disc disorders.

EXAMINATION

Treatment:
Conservative Treatment
Spontaneous improvement of low back discomfort expected within 6 weeks in most of the cases.
Conservative treatments are essentially efforts to reduce inflammation; therefore, only a very short period of rest is appropriate, anti-inflammatories are of some benefit and warm, moist heat or modalities may be helpful. Activities should be resumed as early as tolerated.
Injections (e.g., epidural) may be particularly helpful in patients with radiculopathy by providing symptom relief, which allows the patient to increase activities and helps facilitate rehabilitation

Surgical treatment
Various surgical procedures have been reported and share the common goal of decompressing the neural elements to relieve the leg pain. The most common procedure for a herniated or ruptured intervertebral disk is a microdiscectomy, in which a small incision is made, aided by an operating microscope, and a hemilaminotomy is performed to remove the disk fragment that is impinging on the nerves.

What are red flags symptoms in back pain?

Red flags are symptoms that can indicate a serious problem requiring urgent management:
1. Age of onset less than 20 yrs or more than 55 yrs.
2. Recent history of violent trauma.
3. Constant progressive, non-mechanical pain (no relief with bed rest).
4. Thoracic pain.
5. Past medical history of malignant tumour.
6. Prolonged use of corticosteroids.
7. Drug abuse, immunosuppression, HIV
8. Systematically unwell
9. Unexplained weight loss
10. Widespread neurological symptoms (including cauda equine syndrome)
11. Structural deformity
12. Fever

If the patient develops saddle anaesthesia and incontinence, what is the possible diagnosis, mention other clinical findings and how would you manage it?

Cauda equina syndrome is the most likely diagnosis which results from terminal spinal nerve root compression in the lumbosacral region
Sign and symptoms:
Severe back pain
Saddle anesthesia, i.e., anesthesia or paraesthesia involving S3 to S5 dermatomes, including the perineum, external genitalia and anus.
Bladder and bowel dysfunction, caused by decreased tone of the urinary and anal sphincters.
Sciatica-type pain on one side or both sides, although pain may be wholly absent.
Weakness of the muscles of the lower legs (often paraplegia)
Achilles (ankle) reflex absent on both sides.
Sexual dysfunction.
Absent anal reflex and bulbocavernosus reflex
Gait disturbance
Severe back pain, saddle anesthesia, incontinence and sexual dysfunction are considered "red flags", i.e. features which require urgent treatment.

EXAMINATION

The next step is confirming the diagnosis with urgent MRI. Cauda equina syndrome is regarded as a surgical emergency. Surgical decompression by means of laminectomy or other approaches may be undertaken within 24 - 48 hours of symptoms developing.

What risks does a discectomy carry?

1. Vascular injury—may occur during attempts at disc removal if curets are allowed to penetrate the anterior longitudinal ligament
2. Nerve root injury—more common with anomalous nerve roots
3. Failed back syndrome—often the result of poor patient selection; other causes include:
   Recurrent herniation
   Herniation at another level
   Unrecognized lateral stenosis
   Vertebral instability
   Epidural fibrosis occurs at about 3 months postoperatively and may be associated with back or leg pain.
   It responds poorly to re-exploration. Scarring can be differentiated from recurrent HNP with a gadolinium-enhanced MRI.
4. Dural tear—1% to 4% incidence
5. Wound infection (approximately 1% in open discectomy)
6. Discitis (3-6 weeks postoperatively, with rapid onset of severe back pain)
7. Cauda equina syndrome—secondary to extruded disc, surgical trauma, and hematoma

How would you classify lumbar disc herniation?

Lumbar disc herniation can be classified based on either the location in the vertebral foramen in which the disc herniates or the anatomical part of the disc that herniates as follows:

A. Location classification
Central prolapse: often associated with back pain only, may present with cauda equina syndrome which is a surgical emergency
Posterolateral (paracentral): most common (90-95%) (where the posterior longitudinal ligament is the weakest), affects the traversing/descending/lower nerve root, for example at L4/5 affects L5 nerve root foraminal (far lateral, extraforaminal): less common (5-10%), affects exiting/upper nerve root, for example at L4/5 affects L4 nerve root

B. Anatomic classification
Protrusion: eccentric bulging with an intact annulus.
Extrusion: disc material herniates through annulus but remains continuous with disc space sequestered fragment (free) : disc material herniates through annulus and is no longer continuous with disc space.

Where the spinal cord ends, define conus medularis, filum terminale and cauda equine?

Spinal cord extends from brainstem to inferior border of L1. Conus medullaris is termination of spinal cord. Filum terminale is residual fragment of spinal cord that extends from conus medullaris to sacrum.
Cauda equine is a collection of L1-S5 peripheral nerves within the lumbar canal and filum terminale surrounded by dura that extend from the spinal cord.

What are the important differences between cervical and lumbar nerves?

1. Pedicle/nerve root mismatch for example: cervical spine C6 nerve root travels under C5 pedicle (mismatch) while lumbar spine L5 nerve root travels under L5 pedicle (match)

2. Extra C8 nerve root (no C8 pedicle)

3. horizontal (cervical) vs. vertical (lumbar) anatomy of nerve root. A paracentral and foraminal disc will affect different lumbar nerve roots because of vertical anatomy of the lumbar nerve root while ? will affect the same cervical nerve root because of horizontal anatomy of cervical nerve root.

Describe different parts of lumbar vertebrae?

Components of vertebral bodies:
1. anterior vertebral body
2. posterior arch which is formed by: pedicles and lamina
3. spinous process
4. transverse process
5. mammillary processes: project posteriorly from superior articular facet
6. pars interarticularis: mass of bone between superior and inferior articular facets, site of spondylolysis
7. intervertebral disc: act as an articulation above and below
8. facet joint (zygapophyseal joint): formed by superior and inferior articular processes that project from junction of pedicle and lamina

What is the function of posterior column, lateral spinothalamic tract and lateral corticospinal tract?

Dorsal column is responsible for deep touch, proprioception and vibratory sensation. Lateral spinothalamic tract is responsible for pain and temperature. Lateral corticospinal tract is the main voluntary motor descending tract.

What is the blood supply of the spinal cord and what is the artery of Adamkiewicz?

Spinal cord blood supply provided by:
1. anterior spinal artery: primary blood supply of anterior 2/3 of spinal cord, including both the lateral corticospinal tract and ventral corticospinal tract
2. posterior spinal artery (right and left): primary blood supply to the dorsal sensory columns
   Artery of Adamkiewicz: the largest anterior segmental artery typically arises from left posterior intercostal artery, which branches from the aorta, significant variation exists and in almost 75% it originates on the left side between the T8 and L1 vertebral segments. It supplies the lower two thirds of the spinal cord via the anterior spinal artery.

Do you know a classification system for muscle weakness for patients with spinal injury?

Muscle Grading System by the American Spinal Injury Association (ASIA)
0 Total paralysis

1 Palpable or visible contraction
2 Active movement, full range of motion, gravity eliminated
3 Active movement, full range of motion, against gravity
4 Active movement, full range of motion, against gravity and provides some resistance

EXAMINATION

5 Active movement, full range of motion, against gravity and provides normal resistance
NT Patient unable to reliably exert effort or muscle unavailable for testing due to factors such as immobilization, pain on effort or contracture.

Define scoliosis, mention the most common cause of it, how could you tell the difference between a compensatory, postural and structural scoliosis?

Scoliosis is a lateral curvature of the spine. The commonest cause is a protective scoliosis secondary to a prolapsed intervertebral disc.
Compensatory scoliosis for example in shortened legs which disappears when the patient sits.
Postural scoliosis occurs most frequently in adolescent girls and resolves spontaneously. It is not associated with hump when the patient bends forward.
Structural scoliosis is alteration in vertebral shape and mobility. It does not disappear on sitting and is associated with a hump when bending forward.
A true structural scoliosis may be:
1. Idiopathic (the commonest).
2. Congenital (e.g. hemivertebra, fused vertebra)
3. Paralytic (e.g. polio)
4. Neuropathic (e.g. neurofibromatosis, cerebral palsy)
5. Myopathy (e.g. muscular dystrophy)
6. Metabolic (rickets).

SUMMARY OF EXAMINATION

Wash Your Hands
Ensure that you are seen by the examiners to wash your hands using alcohol gel provided.

Introduce, Explain, Expose and Inspect
Begin by introducing yourself, explain what you are going to do and check that this is OK with the patient and that he/she is not in any pain.
For back examination the patient should be exposed to their underwear.

Patient Standing
Ask the patient to stand and observe for any obvious deformity in the back.

Inspect
Look (from the front, back and sides) for the followings: any obvious deformity (e.g. scoliosis, kyphosis), swellings, scars, abnormal pigmentation like café au lait spots and muscle wasting.

Palpate
For any tenderness over the spine, paraspinal muscles, sacroiliac joints and for any step.

Movements
Forward flexion, Extension, Lateral flexion and rotation

Patient Supine
Ask the patient to lie on the examination couch.
Straight leg raising test, contralateral leg raising test. Complete the examination with full neurological examination including: knee and Achilles reflexes, dermatome and motor examination.

Closing

Thank the patient. Inform them that they may now get dressed or ensure they are adequately covered.

Present your findings to the examiner.

TOP TIPS

➕ The commonest site of disc herniation is L4/L5 and L5/S1 with L5 nerve root and S1 nerve root affected respectively.

➕ When doing straight leg raising test ask about where does it hurt, and confirm the test by dorsiflexing the foot and then bend the knee until pain disappears.

➕ Remember to mention examination of perianal and genital sensation, anal reflexes is part of neurological examination.

References:

1. Reynolds RM1, Browning GG, Nawroz I, Campbell IW. Von Recklinghausen's neurofibromatosis: neurofibromatosis type 1.Lancet. 2003 May 3;361(9368):1552-4.

EXAMINATION

1.16 Shoulder

Scenario

A 40 year old man complains of right shoulder pain for 9 months. The pain is often worsened by shoulder overhead movement and sometimes occurs at night, especially if the patient is lying on the affected shoulder. The patient had a cortisone injection in his right shoulder two months ago resulting in a short period of pain relief.

The patient is comfortable, you have washed you hands, introduced yourself and explained what you are going to do. Please examine this gentleman's shoulder.

Describe how you would begin

Expose and Inspect: Adequate patient exposure, ideally with blouse / shirt off. First ask the patient to walk away a few steps, turn around and come back, whilst checking for normal arm swing.
Look from front, back and side
Skin: Scars, bruising/skin changes, swelling.
Muscle: Asymmetry, deformity (winging of the scapula, wasting of deltoid).
Bone & Joint: Position of both shoulders (dislocations).

🖉 Inspection Findings

The shoulder looks normal without sign of muscle atrophy, scar or any obvious deformity.

Having inspected what would you do next?

Next steps are feel, move and specific tests.

A. Feel (palpation): (Ask about pain before you palpate)
Standing in front of the patient: Feel for temperature, tenderness or crepitus. Start at the sternoclavicular joint, feel along the line of the clavicle and around acromioclavicular joint. Feel around the glenohumeral joint and scapula. Feel trapezius, deltoid and infraspinatus. Extend the shoulder, feel supraspinatus and then the biciptal groove. The biceps tendon may be felt in this position by internally and externally rotating the humerus.
Standing Behind the patient: Check interscapular area for pain, feel for rotator cuff defects
Palpate supraclavicular area for lymphadenopathy.

B. Move:
Active then Passive movements. Feel for crepitus during passive movements.
Movements should be repeated with the scapula stabilized.
Abduction and external rotation: Ask the patient to put their hands behind their head, pushing their elbows back. This is a good screening test for global active shoulder movement.
Adduction and internal rotation: Ask the patient to put their hands behind their back, thumbs pointing to the ceiling. The thumbs should normally reach T6. This is a good screening test for global active shoulder movement.
Flexion (0-180°): Ask the patient to raise their arms forwards, up over their head.
Extension (0-60°): Ask the patient to straighten their arms behind them as far as possible.

Abduction (0-180°): Ask the patient to move their arms away from the side of their body until their hands are touching.
Adduction (0-45°): Ask the patient to cross their arms over the front of their body.
External Rotation (0-90°): Ask the patient to externally rotate their shoulders, keeping their arms tucked into their sides. External rotation may also be tested with the shoulder abducted and elbow flexed.
Internal Rotation: Ask the patient to internally rotate their shoulders, keeping their arms tucked into their sides. Ask the patient to reach up behind their back and touch their opposite scapula. The thumbs should normally reach T6. Internal rotation may also be tested with the shoulder abducted and elbow flexed (0-90°).

C. Specific tests:

1. **Lift-off (Gerber's) test:** Position the patient's hand behind their back, with the dorsum of their hand touching their back and elbow flexed to 90°. Ask the patient to lift the dorsum of their hand touching their back against mild resistance. If the patient is unable to do this without resistance, this indicates subscapularis pathology.

2. **Neer's test:** internally rotate the patient's shoulder and pronate their forearm, keeping arms tucked by their sides. Stabilise the scapula and passively forward flex the shoulder in a continuous movement. If pain is reproduced, this is a positive test for rotator cuff impingement.

3. **Hawkins test:** The patient is examined while sitting with their shoulder flexed to 90° and their elbow flexed to 90°. The examiner grasps and supports proximal to the wrist and elbow to ensure maximal relaxation, the examiner and the patient then quickly rotate the arm internally [4][5]. Pain located below the acromioclavicular joint with internal rotation is considered a positive test result

4. **Apprehension-relocation test:** Ask the patient to lie supine on the examination couch, shoulder joint at the edge of the bed. Abduct the patient's shoulder to 90°. Stabilise and feel the glenohumeral joint with one hand and externally rotate the joint with the other hand. Anterior stability is confirmed as the patient's face becomes apprehensive due to pain (apprehension test). This pain may be relieved with the application of posterior (pushing down towards the couch) pressure to the shoulder (Relocation test). This is positive for anterior stability.
Complete the examination by examining the joint above and below (full neck and elbow examination), check associated lymph nodes and assess distal neurovascular status.

> ### ⟳ Inspection Findings
> The patient has a full range of movement, pain when he abducts the shoulder more than 60°, Hawkins test and Neer test are positive.

Given the history and examination findings this is likely to be impingement syndrome of the right shoulder.

How would you manage this patient?

A. Nonoperative:
Physiotherapy, limit impingement position activity, NSAIDs, subacromial cortisone injection.

B. Operative:
Subacromial decompression (arthroscopic or open).

EXAMINATION

Can you define impingement syndrome and the possible underlying cause(s)?

Shoulder impingement syndrome, also called subacromial impingement, painful arc syndrome, is a clinical syndrome which occurs when there is impingement of the supraspinatus tendon as it passes through the subacromial space, the passage beneath the acromion.

Causes:
When the arm is raised, the subacromial space (gap between the anterior edge of the acromion and the head of the humerus) narrows, through which the supraspinatus muscle tendon passes. Anything that causes further narrowing has the tendency to impinge the tendon and cause an inflammatory response, resulting in impingement syndrome. This can be caused by:
1. Bony structures such as subacromial spurs (bony projections from the acromion), osteoarthritic spurs on the acromioclavicular joint, and variations in the shape of the acromion.
2. Thickening or calcification of the coracoacromial ligament can also cause impingement.
3. Loss of function of the rotator cuff muscles, due to injury or loss of strength, may cause the humerus to move superiorly, resulting in impingement. Inflammation and subsequent thickening of the subacromial bursa may also cause impingement.
4. Idiopathic.

What is the differential diagnosis of a painful shoulder?

1. **Soft tissue:** adhesive capsulitis (frozen shoulder), rotator cuff injury, supraspinatus tendinitis, subacromial bursitis, long head of biceps tendinitis, suprascapular nerve entrapment.
2. **Joint:** Acromioclavicular OA, glenohumeral OA, recurrent dislocation, subluxation.
3. **Referred pain:** cervical spondylosis, cardiac ischemia.
4. **Others:** infection, neoplasm.

What is adhesive capsulitis (frozen shoulder)?

Adhesive capsulitis (frozen shoulder) is a painful and disabling disorder of unclear cause in which the shoulder capsule, the connective tissue surrounding the glenohumeral joint of the shoulder, becomes inflamed and stiff, greatly restricting motion and causing chronic pain. Frozen shoulder is more frequent in diabetic patients and is more severe and more protracted than in the non-diabetic population.
Diagnosis is based on a full history and thorough clinical examination.

How would you treat adhesive capsulitis (frozen shoulder)?

Management of this disorder focuses on restoring joint movement and reducing shoulder pain, involving medications, physical therapy, and/or surgical intervention. Treatment may continue for months, there is no strong evidence to favour any particular approach. Medications frequently used include NSAIDs; corticosteroids are used in some cases either through local injection or systemically. Manual therapists like osteopaths, chiropractors and physiotherapists may include massage therapy and daily extensive stretching. If these measures are unsuccessful, manipulation of the shoulder under general anesthesia to break up the adhesions is sometimes used.

What are structures that contribute to glenohumeral stability?

A. Static restraints
1. Glenohumeral ligaments.

2. Glenoid labrum.
3. Articular congruity and version.

B. Dynamic restraints
Rotator cuff muscles

Can you describe the blood supply of the humeral head?

A. Ascending branch of anterior humeral circumflex artery and arcuate artery.
B. Arcuate artery is the interosseous continuation of the ascending branch of anterior
   humeral circumflex artery and penetrates the bone of the humeral head
C. Posterior humeral circumflex artery: the main blood supply to the humeral head.

Can you describe calcific tendinitis?

Calcific tendonitis refers to a build-up of calcium in the rotator cuff. When calcium builds up in the tendon, it can cause a build up of pressure in the tendon, as well as causing chemical irritation.
This leads to pain. The pain can be extremely intense. It is one of the worst pains in the shoulder.
In addition to the chemical irritation and pressure, the calcific (calcium) deposit reduces the space between the rotator cuff and the acromion, as well as affecting the normal function of the rotator cuff.
This can lead to subacromial impingement between the acromion and the calcium deposit in the rotator cuff when lifting the arm overhead.
The cause of the calcium build-up in the rotator cuff is not known. It tends to be more common in people between the ages of 30-60 years of age.

What is the mechanism of injury in traumatic anterior shoulder instability and what are the most common associated injuries?

Mechanism is an anteriorly directed force on the arm when the shoulder is abducted and externally rotated.
Associated injuries:
1. **Bankart lesion:** is an avulsion of the anterior labrum and anterior band of the inferior glenohumeral ligament from the anterior inferior glenoid.
2. **Hill Sachs defect:** is a chondral impaction injury in the posterosuperior humeral head secondary to contact with the glenoid rim.
3. **Bony Bankart lesion:** is a fracture of the anterior inferior glenoid
4. **Greater tuberosity fracture:** is associated with anterior dislocation in patients > 50 years of age
5. **Lesser tuberosity fracture:** is associated with posterior dislocations
6. **Axillary nerve injury:** is most often a transient neurapraxia of the axillary nerve
7. **Rotator cuff tears:**
    30% of patients > 40 years of age
    80% of patients > 60 years of age

Can you describe rotator cuff muscles and their function?

Rotator cuff is a group of muscles and their tendons that act to stabilize the shoulder. The four muscles are the supraspinatus muscle, the infraspinatus muscle, teres minor muscle, and the subscapularis muscle.

Muscle	Origin on scapula	Attachment on humerus	Function	Innervation

EXAMINATION

1. Supraspinatus	Supraspinatus fossa	Greater tubercle	Abduction	Suprascapular nerve (C5)
2. Infraspinatus	Infraspinatus fossa	Greter tubercle	External rotation	Suprascapular nerve (C5-C6)
3. Teres minor	lateral border	Greater tubercle	External rotation	Axillary nerve (C5)
4. Subscapularis	Subscapular fossa	Lesser tubercle	Internal rotation	Upper and Lower subscapular nerve (C5-C6)

Can you describe rotator cuff arthropathy?

Rotator cuff tears can lead to arthropathy as loss of joint congruence results in abnormal glenohumeral wear leading to the development of a specific pattern of degenerative joint disease.

Rotator cuff arthropathy is defined as a combination of:
1. Massive chronic rotator cuff tear
2. Glenohumeral osteoarthritis

SUMMARY OF EXAMINATION

Wash Your Hands
Ensure that you are seen by the examiners to wash your hands using alcohol gel provided.

Introduce, Explain, Expose and Inspect
Begin by introducing yourself, explain what you are going to do and check that this is OK with the patient and that he/she is not in any pain.
For shoulder examination the patient should ideally be with blouse / shirt off.

Look
Inspect for any scars, swelling, symmetry, deformity and muscle wasting.

Feel
Palpate systematically for any tenderness over the bony structures and soft tissue.

Move (active then passive)
Abduction (initiation, painful arc, ability to hold arm up)
Adduction (hand on opposite shoulder).
Forward (flexion).
Backwards (extension).
Hands behind back (internal rotation).
Hands behind head.
Elbows by side (external rotation, internal rotation).
Elbows abducted (external rotation, internal rotation).
Feel for crepitation.

Specific tests
Test for subscapularis (lift off test (Gerber´s test)).
Test for anterior instability (apprehension/relocation test).
Tests for impingement syndrome (Hawkins test, Neer test).

Closing

Thank the patient. Inform them that they may now get dressed or ensure they are adequately covered.

Present your findings to the examiner.

TOP TIPS

✚ Examine active movements first then passive.

✚ Remember to compare each side, starting with good side first.

✚ Complete the examination by examining the distal neurovascular status.

EXAMINATION

1.17 Hand

Scenario

A 60 year old male farm labourer has gradually developed painless bilateral contractures of his ring fingers. This deformity has begun to affect his ability to do his job. Both his father and brother developed the same deformity, which ended up in surgical intervention. He takes no regular medications. He doesn't smoke or drink alcohol.

The patient is comfortable; you have washed your hands, introduced yourself and explained what you are going to do. Please examine this gentleman's hand.

Describe how you would begin

Expose and Inspect: Sit the patient opposite you, with hands resting on a table / supported by a pillow.
Expose the patient's arm to the elbows bilaterally.
Look for:
Any aids e.g. splints
Scars (trauma, postoperative e.g. carpal tunnel syndrome),
Trophic changes (i.e. increased hair growth or altered sweat production) can represent derangement of sympathetic nervous system.
Deformity (asymmetry, angulation, rotation).
Finger rotational deformity (flex finger against palm, finger tips normally point toward scaphoid – malalignment suggests fracture with rotation).
Erythema.
Muscle wasting.

> #### ⌒ Inspection Findings
>
> There is bilateral flexion deformity of the ring fingers at metacarpophalangeal (MCP) and proximal Interphalangeal (PIP) joints. There is no scar, erythema or muscle wasting.

Having inspected what would you do next?

Next steps are feel, move and specific tests.

A. Feel (palpation): (Ask about pain before you palpate)
Tenderness: palpate each joint separately and systematically. Check the anatomical snuffbox for
tenderness that may be associated with a scaphoid fracture, particularly in the acute setting.
Palmar fascia thickening (Dupuytren´s contracture).
Rheumatoid nodules: subcutaneous lesions, usually on extensor surfaces.
Hand nerves: screen for the following nerve injuries, by assessing fine touch. If an injury is suspected,
perform a thorough nerve examination.
1. Radial nerve: first dorsal web space.
2. Median nerve: thenar eminence.
3. Ulnar nerve: palmar aspect of little finger.

EXAMINATION

B. Move:
Active then Passive movements. Feel for crepitus during passive movements.
Movements should be compared with the other hand.

General functional assessment:
Flex thumb, make a fist and fan out fingers, abduct and adduct fingers, power grip.

Range of motion:
Thumb:
CMC palmar adduction/abduction: contact/45°.
CMC radial adduction/abduction: contact/60°.
CMC opposition: tip of thumb to base or tip of fifth digit.
Thumb MCP: extension/flexion (10°/55°).
Thumb IP: extension/flexion (15°/80°).
Fingers:
MCP: extension/flexion (0°/85°).
PIP: extension/flexion (0°/110°).
DIP: extension/flexion (0°/65°).
Wrist:
Wrist extension: 70°.
Wrist flexion: 90°.
Wrist radial deviation: 20°.
Wrist ulnar deviation: 50°.
Pronation / supination: 80° / 85°.

Digital tendons: test continuity of the tendons, inability to assume position of function is a red flag.
Thumb
FPL: flex IP against resistance.
EPL: patient keeps palmar surface of hand flat on a table and lifts thumb.
Digital flexors
FDP: MCP + PIP joints held in extension while patient asked to flex FDP, thereby isolating FDP (from FDS) as the only tendon capable of flexing the finger.
FDS: MCP, PIP and DIP of all fingers held in extension with hand flat and palm up; the finger to be tested is then allowed to flex at PIP joint
Digital extensors
EDC: extension against resistance
Extensor indicis and extensor digiti minimi: tested together by asking the patient to make a fist and extend their index and little fingers.

C. Specific tests:

1. **Tinnel's test:** Take the patient's hand, palmar surface up. Tap their forearm, proximal to distal, along the course of the median nerve. Ensure that tapping is extended over the region of the carpal tunnel, which may reproduce carpal tunnel syndrome symptoms e.g. tingling.

2. **Phalen's test:** Ask the patient to hold their wrist in complete and forced flexion, pushing the dorsal surface of both hands together for 1 minute. This compresses the median nerve as it runs through the carpal tunnel such that reproduction of carpal tunnel syndrome symptoms may occur.

3. **Finkelstein's test:** Ask the patient to flex the thumb, form a fist over it, then ulnar deviate the wrist. This may reproduce symptoms of De Quervian's tenosynovitis.

4. **Froment's sign:** tests for ulnar nerve motor weakness. Ask the patient to hold a piece

EXAMINATION

of paper between thumb and radial side of index. Test is positive if, as the paper is pulled away by the examiner, the patient flexes the thumb IP joint in an attempt to hold onto paper

Brief Neurologic Examination

Ulnar Nerve
Finger abduction against resistance
Sensation to ulnar 1.5 fingers on palmar aspect (e.g. tip of pinky finger)
Median Nerve
Sensation to radial 3.5 fingers and dorsal tips (e.g. tip of index finger).
Oppose thumb to index finger against resistance.
Radial Nerve
Wrist extension (dorsiflexion) against resistance
Sensation to dorsal first 3.5 fingers (e.g. dorsal first web space)
Fine functional assessment: pick up a key (pincer grip). Unbutton and button shirt. Pick up a pen and write a short sentence.

Two-point discrimination test
Normal <6mm.
Fair: 6 -10 mm.
Poor: 11 -16 mm

Complete the examination by examining joints above (full wrist and elbow examination), check associated lymph nodes and assess upper limb neurovascular status (radial pulse, ulnar pulse, Allen's test, capillary refill).

> ### ⌒ Findings
> The patient has painless, bilateral nodular thickening of the palm extending distally to involve the ring and little fingers.

Given the history and examination findings, this is Dupuytren's contracture.

What else would you like to examine?

I would like to examine the sole of the feet (can affect the plantar aponeurosis), the liver (alcoholism is associated with Dupuytren's contracture and can produce a large fatty liver), the dorsal knuckle pads and the penis (fibrosis of the corpus cavernosum causing curvature of the penis, Peyronie's disease).

Can you describe Dupuytren's contracture and the associated risk factors?

Dupuytren's contracture is a fibrosing disorder that results in slowly progressive thickening and shortening of the palmar fascia and leads to debilitating digital contractures, particularly of MCP joints or the proximal interphalangeal (PIP) joints. Dupuytren's contracture is most commonly observed in persons of northern european descent. Many individuals have bilateral disease (45%); in unilateral cases, the right side is more often affected. The ring finger is most commonly involved, followed by the fifth digit and then the middle finger.
Although the cause of Dupuytren's disease is unknown, a family history is often present. Males are three times as likely to develop disease and are more likely to have higher disease severity.
Other potential risk factors include manual labour with vibration exposure, prior hand

trauma, alcoholism, smoking, diabetes mellitus, hyperlipidemia, Peyronie's disease, and complex regional pain syndrome.

Can you name conditions that are related to Dupuytren's contracture?

1. Peyronie's disease – curvature of the penis.
2. Ledderhose's disease – Plantar fibromatosis, callus under the foot and possible curling under of toes.
3. Garrod's pad – pads on the back of knuckles of fingers.
4. Frozen shoulder – shoulder that develops stiffness and limited range of motion.

How would you manage this patient?

A. Nonoperative
Range of motion exercises, early efficacy seen with injections of clostridial collagenase into Dupuytren's cords causes lysis and rupture of cords
B. Operative
surgical resection/fasciectomy
Indications:
MCP flexion contractures > 30°
PIP flexion contractures

What are the complications of operative treatment?

1. Hematoma
2. Recurrence
3. Flare reaction: pain syndrome with diffuse swelling, hyperesthesia, redness and stiffness increased risk with concomitant carpal tunnel release
4. Neurovascular injury: bundle at risk due to central and superficial displacement from spiral cord, identify prior to excising cord.

Can you describe nerve conduction studies, types and indications?

Nerve Conduction Studies comprises nerve conduction velocity (NCV) studies and electromyography (EMG) used to:
localize areas of compression and neuropathy
distinguish lower vs upper motor neuron lesions (spinal root, trunk, division, cord or peripheral nerve lesion).
determine severity and prognosis (neuropraxia has good prognosis while axonotmesis/neurotmesis has poor prognosis
demonstrate denervation, reinnervation
Indications:
carpal tunnel syndrome
cubital tunnel syndrome
cervical radiculopathy
lumbar radiculopathy
nerve dysfunction of the shoulder (e.g., scapular winging)

Describe the following deformities: Swan neck, Boutonnière and Mallet finger deformity?

Boutonniere Deformity
Characterized by:
PIP flexion and DIP extension.

Mechanism:
Caused by rupture of the central slip over PIP joint from laceration, traumatic avulsion, capsular distension in rheumatoid arthritis. Rupture of central slip causes the extrinsic extension mechanism from the EDC to be lost which prevents extension at the PIP joint. Attenuation of triangular ligament causes intrinsic muscles of the hand (lumbricals) to act as flexors at the PIP joint. Lumbricals also extend the DIP joint without an opposing or balancing force.

Swan Neck Deformity
Characterized by:
hyperextension of PIP and flexion of DIP.
Mechanism:
Caused by lax volar plate, imbalance of muscle forces on PIP (extension force > flexion force).

Mallet finger deformity
Characterized by:
A finger deformity caused by disruption of the terminal extensor tendon distal to DIP joint, the disruption may be bony or tendinous.
Mechanism:
Traumatic impaction blow which is usually caused by a traumatic impaction blow (i.e. sudden forced flexion) to the tip of the finger in the extended position.
Dorsal laceration to the dorsal DIP joint which is a less common mechanism of injury.

Can you describe carpal tunnel syndrome (CTS)?

It is a medical condition in which the median nerve is compressed as it travels through the wrist at the carpal tunnel. It is the most common compressive neuropathy.
Presentation:
Symptoms:
numbness and tingling in radial 3-1/2 digits
clumsiness
pain and paraesthesia that awaken patient at night
Physical exam:
inspection may show thenar atrophy
carpal tunnel compression test (Durkan's test): is the most sensitive test to diagnose carpal tunnel syndrome. Performed by pressing thumbs over the carpal tunnel and holding pressure for 30 seconds.
Onset of pain or paresthesia in the median nerve distribution within 30 seconds is a positive result.
Phalen's test (see above).
Tinnel's test (see above).

How would you treat a patient with CTS?

Treatment:
A. Nonoperative
NSAIDS, night splints, activity modifications, steroid injection.

B. Operative
Carpal tunnel release
Indications
Failure of nonoperative treatment (including steroid injections).
Acute CTS following a distal radius fracture.

Can you mention the fingers (dig 2-5) flexors, extensors and their nerve supply?

A.   Fingers flexors:
1. **Flexor Digitorum Superficialis (FDS)**
   Action: Flexes PIP joints of digits 2-5.
   Innervation: Median nerve.
2. **Flexor Digitorum Profundus(FDP)**
   Action: Flexes DIP joints of digits 2-5.
   Innervation: Medial part: ulnar nerve (C8 and T1); Lateral part: anterior interosseous branch of median nerve.

B. Fingers extensors:
1. **Extensor Digitorum**
   Action: Extends MCP joints of digits 2-5.
   Innervation: Posterior interosseous nerve (branch of the radial nerve).
2. **Extensor Digiti Minimi**
   Action: Extends 5th digit at MCP and interphalangeal joints.
   Innervation: Posterior interosseous nerve (branch of the radial nerve).
3. **Extensor Indicis**
   Action: Extends 2nd digit at MCP and interphalangeal joints.
   Innervation: Posterior interosseous nerve (branch of the radial nerve).

Can you describe muscles of the thumb and their nerve supply?

1. **Flexor Pollicis Longus**
   Action: Flexes IP joint of the thumb.
   Innervation: Anterior interosseous nerve from median nerve.
2. **Extensor Pollicis Longus**
   Action: Extends IP joint of the thumb.
   Innervation: Posterior interosseous nerve (branch of the radial nerve).
3. **Extensor Pollicis Brevis**
   Action: Extends PIP joint of the thumb.
   Innervation: Posterior interosseous nerve (branch of the radial nerve).
4. **Thenar muscles:**
A. **Opponens Pollicis**
   Action: Draws 1st metacarpal laterally to oppose thumb toward center of palm and rotates it medially.
   Innervation: Recurrent branch of median nerve.
B. **Abductor Pollicis Brevis**
   Action: Abducts thumb and helps oppose it.
   Innervation: Recurrent branch of median nerve.
C. **Flexor Pollicis Brevis**
   Action: Flexes thumb.
   Innervation: Recurrent branch of median nerve.
D. **Adductor Pollicis**
   Action: Adducts thumb.
   Innervation: Deep branch of ulnar nerve.

Can you describe the intrinsic muscles of the hand and their nerve supply?

1. **Dorsal interossei**
   Action: Abduct digits from axial line and act with lumbricals to flex MCP joints and extend IP joints
   Innervation: Deep branch of ulnar nerve.
2. **Palmar interossei**

EXAMINATION

Action: Adduct digits toward axial line and act with lumbricals to flex MCP joints and extend IP joints.
Innervation: Deep branch of ulnar nerve.
3. **Lumbrical Muscles**
Action: Extends PIP and DIP joint.
Innervation:
1nd & 2nd lumbricals innervated by median nerve.
3rd & 4th lumbricals innervated by ulnar nerve.

Can you describe the nerve supply of the hand?

The hand is innervated by 3 nerves: the median, ulnar, and radial. Each has sensory and motor components.

A. Median nerve
The median nerve is responsible for innervating the muscles involved in the fine precision and pinch function of the hand.
It originates from the lateral and medial cords of the brachial plexus (C5-T1).
In the forearm, the motor branches supply the pronator teres, flexor carpi radialis, palmaris longus, and FDS muscles. The anterior interosseous branch innervates the flexor pollicis longus, FDP (index and long finger), and pronator quadratus muscles.
Proximal to the wrist, the palmar cutaneous branch provides sensation at the thenar eminence.
As the median nerve passes through the carpal tunnel, the recurrent motor branch innervates the thenar muscles (abductor pollicis brevis, opponens pollicis, and superficial head of flexor pollicis brevis).
It also innervates the index and long finger lumbrical muscles.
Sensory digital branches provide sensation to the thumb, index, long, and radial side of the ring finger.

B. Ulnar nerve
The ulnar nerve is responsible for innervating the muscles involved in the power grasping function of the hand.
It originates at the medial cord of the brachial plexus (C8-T1).
Motor branches innervate the flexor carpi ulnaris and FDP muscles to the ring and small fingers.
Proximal to the wrist, the palmar cutaneous branch provides sensation at the hypothenar eminence.
The dorsal **branch, which branches from** the main trunk at the distal forearm, provides sensation to the ulnar portion of the dorsum of the hand and small finger, and part of the ring finger.
At the hand, the superficial branch forms the digital nerves, which provide sensation at the small finger and ulnar aspect of the ring finger. The deep motor branch passes through the Guyon canal in company with the ulnar artery. It innervates the hypothenar muscles (abductor digiti minimi, opponens digiti minimi, flexor digiti minimi, and palmaris brevis), all interossei, the 2 ulnar lumbricals, the adductor pollicis, and the deep head of the flexor pollicis brevis.

C. Radial nerve
The radial nerve is responsible for innervating the wrist extensors, which control the position of the hand and stabilize the fixed unit.
It originates from the posterior cord of the brachial plexus (C6-8).
At the elbow, motor branches innervate the brachioradialis and extensor carpi radialis longus muscles.
At the proximal forearm, the radial nerve divides into the superficial and deep branches. The deep posterior interosseous branch innervates all the muscles in the extensor compartment: supinator, extensor carpi radialis brevis, extensor digitorum communis,

extensor digiti minimi, extensor carpi ulnaris, extensor indicis, extensor pollicis longus, extensor pollicis brevis, and abductor pollicis longus.

The superficial branch provides sensation at the radial aspect of the dorsum of the hand, the dorsum of the thumb, and the dorsum of the index finger, long finger, and radial half of the ring finger proximal to the distal interphalangeal joints.

How can you classify peripheral nerve injury and mention prognosis for each type?

The most used classification systems for classifying peripheral nerve injury are: the Seddon and the Sunderland classification.

A. Seddon Classification
1. Neuropraxia: nerve contusion leading to reversible conduction block without Wallerian degeneration.
 Recovery prognosis is excellent.
2. Axonotmesis: axon and myelin sheath disruption leads to conduction block with Wallerian degeneration, endoneurium remains intact.
3. Neurotmesis: complete nerve division with disruption of endoneurium. No recovery unless surgical repair performed

Sunderland Classification
1st degree
same as neuropraxia
2nd degree
same as axonotmesis
3rd degree
injury with endoneurial scarring
4th degree
nerve in continuity but at the level of injury there is complete scarring across the nerve
5th degree
same as neurotmesis

SUMMARY OF EXAMINATION

Wash Your Hands
Ensure that you are seen by the examiners to wash your hands using alcohol gel provided.

Introduce, Explain, Expose and Inspect
Begin by introducing yourself, explain what you are going to do and check that this is OK with the patient and that he/she is not in any pain.
For hand examination the patient should ideally be exposed to elbows bilaterally.

Look
Inspect for any scars, swelling, symmetry, deformity and muscle wasting.

Feel
Palpate systematically for any tenderness over the bony structures and soft tissue.

Move (active then passive)
Flex thumb, make a fist and fan out fingers, abduct and adduct fingers, power grip.

EXAMINATION

Specific tests
1. **Tinnel's test**
2. **Phalen's test**
3. **Finkelstein test**
4. **Froment's sign**

Closing
Thank the patient. Inform them that they may now get dressed or ensure they are adequately covered.
Present your findings to the examiner.

TOP TIPS

➕ Examine active movements first then passive.

➕ Look for muscle wasting at thenar / hypothenar eminence, dorsal intermetacarpal wasting.

➕ Remember to compare each side, starting with good side first.

➕ Complete the examination by examining the distal neurovascular status.

1.18 | Hip

Scenario

A 66 year old male complains of right groin pain for two years. The patient describes the pain as aching in nature, mostly after overuse or long periods of inactivity. He cannot go long distances as he used to before.

The patient is comfortable, you have washed your hands, introduced yourself and explained what you are going to do. Please examine this gentleman's hip.

Describe how you would begin

Expose and Inspect: Adequate patient exposure, ideally to underwear. This is to assist examination of the joint above (spine) and below (knee). Comment on use of aids e.g. stick, frame, brace etc.

A. Standing position:
From the front: pelvic tilting, muscle wasting, scars.
From the side: increase in lumbar lordosis.
From behind: scoliosis, gluteal muscle wasting.
You can do Trendelenburg´s test already here (see later in the chapter).
B. Lying position: inspect for any apparent leg length discrepancy.

> ### 👓 Inspection Findings
> The right limb is 1 cm shorter and there is mild gluteal muscle wasting. There are no scars.

Having inspected what would you do next?

Next steps are feel, move and specific tests.

A. Feel (palpation): By palpation you are looking for the following (ask about pain before you palpate):
1. Pain:
   A. Palpate the hip joint, which lies deep to the femoral artery, at the mid-inguinal ligament.
   B. Greater trochanter: palpated laterally.
   C. Adductor longus: palpate medially along the entire length.
   D. Ischial tuberosity: turn the patient on their side to palpate the ischial tuberosity.

2. Crepitus: by rotating the limb medially and laterally.

3. Assess apparent shortening: Measure the true length and the apparent length. Check that anterior superior iliac spines (ASIS) are parallel. Heels should now be level. Measure ASIS to medial malleolus for true length, xiphisternum to medial malleolus for apparent length.
   If there is any discrepancy you should flex the knees and see if the shortening is located in the femur or the tibia. Shortening in the femoral shaft is demonstrated as the knee of the affected limb lies proximal-inferior to the knee of the contra-lateral limb. Shortening in the tibia is demonstrated as the the knee of the affected limb lies distal-inferior to the knee of the contra-lateral limb.

Put heels together and flex knees to 90°. If the knee of the short leg is proximal to the contra-lateral knee, the femur is short. If it is distal, the tibia is shortened. This can be confirmed by measuring from the tibial tubercle to the medial malleolus.

4. Lymphadenopathy: assess inguinal lymph nodes.

B. Move:
1. Flexion and extension:
   Extension is tested with the patient lying prone or on their side. Fix the pelvis by putting your hand on the back, lift each straight leg separately. Extension can be tested by the Thomas test also (see later in the chapter).
   Flexion is tested using one hand under the pelvis to check no further movement occurs, and with the opposite hip held by the patient in enough flexion to obliterate lumbar lordosis. Normal range is about 120° and the thigh should touch the abdomen.
2. Abduction and adduction:
   You have to put your hand over the ASIS to make sure the pelvis is fixed.
   Abduction is tested by asking the patient how far he/she can bring the examined leg out (normal range is about 40°).
   Adduction is tested by asking the patient how far they can swing the examined leg over the other leg (normal range is about 25° and the leg should cross around mid-thigh).
3. Internal and external rotation: there are two ways to examine hip rotation.
   A. Examination of hip rotation in flexion position: Bend the hip and knee to 90°.
   Internal rotation is tested by stabilising the knee and rotating the leg laterally (normal range is 35°).
   External rotation is tested by stabilising the knee and rotating the leg medially (normal range is 45°).
   B. Examination of hip rotation in extension position: is assessed by making the patient lie with legs extended and rolling the leg laterally (external rotation, normal range is about 45°) and medially (internal rotation, normal range is about 35°).

C. Specific tests:
1. Thomas test: Place your hand behind the lumbar spine to assess its position. Flex the contra-lateral hip fully, observing with the hand that the lumbar curvature is fully flattened. Ask the patient to hold the contra-lateral hip in this position. If the hip being examined rises from the couch, this means there is a fixed flexion deformity/loss of extension in this hip.
2. Trendelenburg's test: is performed in standing position. Check that the ASIS are at the same level. Ask the patient to stand on the leg being examined. The patient should keep the pelvis parallel to the floor. If he/she cannot maintain the pelvis in this position i.e. the pelvis is tilted, the test is positive. This indicates weakness of the gluteal medius and minimus muscles at the side of the hip being examined.

D. Completion:
Check the associated lymph nodes, full spine and knee examination, and distal neurovascular status.

👓 Findings

The patient has pain when moving the hip and restricted range of motion mostly internal rotation. Thomas test was positive with 10° fixed flexion deformity and Trendelenburg's test was positive for the right hip. Plain X-ray for the right hip is done and is below:

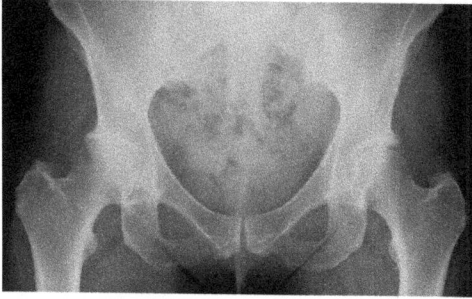

Given the history and examination findings this is likely to be primary OA of the right hip joint.

How would you manage this patient?

A. Nonoperative:
First line treatment for all patients with symptomatic arthritis includes the following: activity modification, physical therapy and weight loss, Paracetamol and NSAIDs. Corticosteroid joint injections can be considered.

B. Operative
1. Arthroscopic debridement: controversial in treatment of degenerative labral tears.
2. Total hip arthroplasty (THA): end-stage, symptomatic or severe osteoarthritis.

What are the causes of shortening of the leg?

1. True shortening: the affected limb is physically shorter than other limb.
   A. Causes distal to the hip joint: growth disturbance (polio, bone or joint infection, epiphyseal trauma). Old femoral or tibial fractures.
   B. Causes in the hip joint: coxa vara (from femoral neck fractures, Perthes´disease, congenital coxa vara), loss of articular joint (infection, arthritis) or dislocation.
2. Apparent lengthening: limb is not altered in length but appears short as a result of an adduction contracture of the hip which has to be compensated for by tilting of the pelvis.

What are the causes for a positive Trendelenburg's test?

1. Gluteal paralysis or weakness.
2. Gluteal inhibition from pain arising in the hip joint.
3. Gluteal insufficiency due to coxa vara which shortens the distance between the origin and insertion of the gluteal muscles.
4. Gluteal insufficiency due to congenital dislocation of the hip.
5. False positive due to pain, generalized weakness, poor cooperation or bad balance.

Name the findings of primary OA of the hip in plain X-ray?

1. joint space narrowing
2. osteophytes
3. subchondral sclerosis
4. subchondral cysts

How many surgical approaches do you know to perform THA and which one is preferable?

1. Posterolateral:
is most common approach for primary and revision arthroplasty, no true interval.
Advantages:
1. Abductor mechanism not violated
2. Good exposure of both femur and acetabulum
3. Easily converted to more extensile exposures both proximally and distally
Disadvantages:
Dislocation rates may be higher than anterior exposures.

2. Direct lateral:
less commonly used approach for arthroplasty, no true interval, splits gluteus medius+/ – vastus lateralis.
Advantages:
1. lower dislocation rate than posterior approach.
2. allows access to both anterior and posterior hip joint without osteotomy.
Disadvantages:
Violates abductor mechanism and may lead to postoperative limp.

3. Anterolateral:
less commonly used approach for arthroplasty, uses interval between tensor fascia lata and gluteus medius.
Advantages:
Lower dislocation rate than posterior approach.
Disadvantages:
Violates abductor mechanism and may lead to postoperative limp.

4. Direct anterior:
increasingly popular approach with good results, uses interval between tensor fascia lata and sartorious.
Advantages:
1. Decreased dislocation rate when compared to posterior approach in numerous studies.
2. Abductor mechanism not violated (compared to anterolateral exposure).
Other eventual advantages include:
decreased muscle damage
decreased pain
quicker recovery
Disadvantages:
1. steep learning curve, complication rates decrease after 100+ procedures.
2. surgical site infection rates increased in obese patients with large abdominal panni.
3. femoral exposure can be challenging.
4. may require a special operating room table for increased exposure.
5. lateral femoral cutaneous nerve paraesthesia.
6. intraoperative fracture rate may be higher.

What are the possible complications following THA?

1. Sciatic nerve palsy.
2. Leg length discrepancy.
3. THA dislocation.
4. Periprosthetic fractures.
5. Periprosthetic infection.
6. Aseptic loosening.
7. Heterotopic ossification.
8. Vascular injury.
9. DVT and PE.

What are the risk factors and commonest microorganism for periprosthetic infection?

Risk factors:
1. Immune suppression: due to
   A. immunosuppressant drugs like: anti-TNF agents, antimetabolites (e.g. methotrexate), corticosteroids.
   B. immunosuppressive conditions (e.g. AIDS)
2. Perioperative surgical site infection.
3. Poor wound healing.
4. Rheumatoid arthritis.
5. Psoriasis.
6. Diabetes.
7. Smoking.
8. Obesity.

Most common organisms include:
1. staphylococcus aureus.
2. staphylococcus epidermidis.
3. Coagulase-negative Staphylococcus (chronic infections).

How do you confirm the diagnosis of periprosthetic infection?

A. Clinical assessment
Acute postoperative infections present with acute onset with swelling, erythema, discharge, warmth, and tenderness.
Chronic infections show pain and more subtle symptoms.

B. Imaging:
Radiographs:
periosteal reaction
scattered patches of osteolysis
Bone scan:
Tc-99m (technetium) detects inflammation and In-111 (indium) detects leukocyte, triple scan can
differentiate infection from fracture or bone remodeling, sensitivity and specificity: 99% sensitivity and
30% to 40% specificity.

C. Studies:
1. Labs:
   WBC
   ESR and CRP
2. Joint aspiration:
   sensitivity 57% to 93% and specificity 88% to 100%.
3. Microbiology:
   definitive diagnosis can be made if the same organism is obtained by repeated aspirations on at least
   three of five periprosthetic specimens obtained at surgery.

What is OA?

a disease of synovial joint, characterized by cartilaginous loss and bony response, resulting in joint
degeneration and destruction.

What are the causes of OA?

A. Primary:
No underlying cause is attributable.
B. Secondary:
1. Congenital: Perthe´s disease.
2. Endocrine: Acromegaly.
3. Infective: osteomyelitis.
4. Inflammatory: RA.
5. Metabolic: Gout.
6. Traumatic: Malunited fractures. Intraarticular fractures.

Name the hip muscles, action and their nerve supply?

1. **Hip Flexors (femoral n.)**
   Iliacus
   Psoas
   Sartorius
   Pectineus
2. **Hip Abductors (gluteal n.)**
   Gluteus maximus (major extensor).
   Gluteus medius (major abductor).
   Gluteus minimus.
3. **Hip Adductors (obturator n.)**
   Adductor longus.
   Adductor brevis.
   Adductor magnus (major adductor).
   Gracilis.
4. **Hip extensors, Hamstring m. (tibial n.)**
   Semitendinosus.
   Semimembranosus.
5. **Hip External Rotators**
   Piriformis (Piriformis nerve (L5, S1, S2).
   Obturator externus (obturator nerve).
   Obturator internus (nerve to obturator n and superior gemellus).
   Superior gemellus (nerve to obturator n and superior gemellus).
   Inferior Gemellus (nerve to the quadratus femoris).
   Quadratus femoris (nerve to the quadratus femoris).

SUMMARY OF EXAMINATION

Wash Your Hands
Ensure that you are seen by the examiners to wash your hands using alcohol gel provided.

Introduce, Explain, Expose and Inspect
Begin by introducing yourself, explain what you are going to do and check that this is OK with the patient and that he/she is not in any pain.

For hip examination the patient should be exposed to underwear.

Look
Inspect both at standing (from the front, back and sides) and in lying position for the followings and observe for any scars, swelling, symmetry, deformity and muscle wasting.

Feel
Palpate systematically for any tenderness over the bony structures and soft tissue. Inspect for any apparent leg length discrepancy.

Move
Flexion and Extension, Adduction and abduction, Internal and external rotation

Specific tests
1. Thomas test
2. Trendelenburg's test

Closing
Thank the patient. Inform them that they may now get dressed or ensure they are adequately covered.
Present your findings to the examiner.

EXAMINATION

TOP TIPS

➕ Movements should ideally be tested actively, passively and against resistance, with the pelvis square.

➕ Remember to compare each side, starting with the good side first.

➕ Start with Thomas' test to unmark fixed flexion deformity.

1.19 | Knee

Scenario

A 26 year old male presents with pain and swelling of his right knee after a twisting injury sustained over the weekend whilst playing rugby league.

The patient is comfortable, you have washed your hands, introduced yourself and explained what you are going to do. Please examine this gentleman's knee.

Describe how you would begin

Expose and Inspect: Adequate patient exposure, ideally to underwear. This is to assist examination of gait, the spine, the hip and the ankle joint.
Look for the following: Do the knees look symmetrical? Look for generalized or localized swelling, bruising, scars, any deformity and quadriceps muscle wasting.

Inspection Findings

The knee looks swollen, bruising over medial side of the knee. There is no scar or muscle wasting. The patient cannot fully extend the knee.

Having inspected what would you do next?

Next steps are feel, move and specific tests.

A. Feel (palpation): By palpation you are looking for the following (ask about pain before you palpate):

Tenderness: Joint line tenderness, tenderness over soft tissue structures (pes anserine bursae, patellar tendon, iliotibial band).

Effusion:
1. **Cross-fluctuation test:** empty the medial compartment superiorly, then empty the suprapatellar pouch inferiorly, and then compress the lateral compartment. Look for fluid transmission across the joint, appearing medially.
2. **Patellar tap test:** empty the suprapatellar pouch inferiorly and then with the index finger of your other hand, push the patella downward, onto the femur. A spring back is positive. This is for moderate effusions.
3. Bulge test: empty the medial compartment superiorly and then compress the lateral compartment. Look for a bulge in the medial compartment. This is for minimal effusion.

Flexion deformity: place your hand under the patient's knee and ask them to push the back of their knee down to the couch. If your hand is compressed, there is no flexion deformity. If there is a gap under the patient's knee when they perform this manoeuver, without hand compression, there is a flexion deformity.

B. Move:
Range of Motion (patient supine)
1. Flexion/Extension: 0° extension to 130° flexion
2. Rotation: varies with flexion; in full extension, there is minimal rotation; at 90° flexion, 45° external rotation and 30° internal rotation.

C. Specific tests:

A. Tests for cruciate ligaments (sagittal stability)

ACL injury test
1. Lachman's test: most sensitive exam test. Performed with 20-30 degrees knee flexion with patient's heel on the couch. Stabilise the patient's thigh with one hand and pull the tibia anteriorly with your other hand. The test is positive if there is anterior tibia translation.

PCL injury test
1. **Posterior sag sign:** patient lies supine with hips and knees flexed to 90°, examiner supports ankles and observes for a posterior shift of the tibia as compared to the uninvolved knee.
2. **Posterior drawer:** with the knee at 90° flexion, a posteriorly directed force is applied to the proximal tibia and posterior tibial translation is quantified.
3. **Quadriceps active test:** attempt to extend a knee flexed at 90° to elicit quadriceps contraction – positive if anterior reduction of the tibia occurs relative to the femur.

B. Tests for collateral ligament injury (coronal stability)

Test the collateral ligaments with 30° knee flexion. Tuck the patient's foot under your arm and stabilize their knee on either side of the joint with both hands. Use a combination of body movement and pressure on the knee to apply valgus (testing the MCL) and varus stress (testing LCL). Repeat collateral ligament tests with 0° knee extension. Varus/valgus deviation in 0° knee extension is always abnormal. **Valgus/varus instability** at 30° only indicates isolated MCL or LCL respectively; while instability at 0° and 30° – combined MCL and ACL and/or PCL

C. Tests for Meniscus injury

1. **McMurray's test:** flex the knee and place a hand on the medial side of knee, externally rotate the leg and bring the knee into extension, a palpable pop or click is a positive test and can correlate with a medial meniscus tear.
2. **Apply compression test:** Testing leg flexed to 90° with patient lying prone on examination table.
   Compression Test
   Lean on patient's foot, applying pressure to heel, compresses tibia into femur, rotate tibia internally and externally on femur, positive compression test suggests meniscal injury.
   Distraction Test
   Kneel gently on back of patient's thigh to stabilize, apply traction to leg pulling tibia from femur, rotate tibia internally and externally. Positive distraction test suggests ligament injury.
3. **Thessaly test:** standing at 20 degrees of knee flexion on the affected limb, the patient twists with knee external and internal rotation with positive test being discomfort or clicking.

D. Tests for Patella instability

Patellar apprehension: Displacing the patella laterally with the thumb, whilst gently flexing the knee may induce pain and laxity. This is a positive test and the patient will resist further movement.

EXAMINATION

> ### 〰️ Findings
> The patient has tenderness on medial side of the knee joint, mild effusion, McMurray's test positive and has 30° extension defect, difficult to examine knee stability because of the pain.

What is your differential diagnosis?

1. Meniscus injury
2. MCL Injury
3. ACL Injury
4. LCL injury
5. Patella dislocation
6. PCL Injury

Given the history and examination findings this is likely to be a medial meniscus injury.

How would you manage this patient?

I would like to confirm my diagnosis by proceeding with investigations as follow:
Plain radiography
Indicated before proceeding with other special tests to rule out skeletal injury. Should be normal in young patients with an acute meniscal injury.
MRI
MRI is most sensitive diagnostic test, but also has false positive findings.

Treatment
The patient's age and locked knee are indications to proceed with operative treatment.

What are the types of operative treatments do you know to treat meniscus injury, mention indication(s) and prognosis for each type?

1. **Partial meniscectomy:**
   Indications:
   Tears not amenable to repair (complex, degenerative, radial tear patterns)
   Predictors of success:
   Age <40 years
   Normal alignment
   Minimal or no arthritis
   Single tear

2. **Meniscal repair**
   Indications:
   1. Peripheral in the red zone (vascularized region). Rim idth is the distance from the tear to the peripheral meniscocapsular junction (blood supply). Rim width correlates with the ability of a meniscal repair to heal (lower rim width has better blood supply)
   2. Vertical and longitudinal tear: 1-4 cm in length
   3. Acute repair combined with ACL reconstruction
   Predictors of success:
   1. Rim width is the distance from the tear to the peripheral meniscocapsular junction (blood supply). Rim width correlates with the ability of a meniscal repair to heal (lower rim width has better blood supply)

2. Highest success when done with concomitant ACL reconstruction
3. Poor results with untreated ACL-deficiency (30%)

Can you mention the complications of meniscus operative treatment?

Complications
1. Saphenous neuropathy (7%)
2. Arthrofibrosis (6%)
3. Sterile effusion (2%)
4. Peroneal neuropathy (1%)
5. Superficial infection (1%)
6. Deep infection (1%)

Can you describe meniscus anatomy, function?

Anatomy:
Medial meniscus: C-shaped with triangular cross section
Lateral meniscus: is more circular (the horns are closer together and approximate the ACL), medial meniscus has less mobility with more rigid peripheral fixation than the lateral meniscus

Function:
1. **Force transmission:** the meniscus functions to optimize force transmission across the knee. It does this by: increasing congruency, increases contact area leading to decreased point loading
2. **Shock-absorption:** the meniscus is more elastic than articular cartilage, and therefore absorbs shock, transmits 50% weight-bearing load in extension, 85% in flexion
3. **Stability:** the meniscus deepens the tibial surface and acts as secondary stabilizer

Can you describe the types of meniscal injury and which meniscus is more susceptible to injury?

Classification of meniscal injury
1. According to location:
A. Red zone (outer third, vascularized)
B. Red-white zone (middle third)
C. White zone (inner third, avascular)
2. According to the size
3. According to the pattern of the injury:
A. Vertical/longitudinal: common, especially with ACL tears, repair when peripheral
B. Bucket handle: vertical tear which may displace into the notch, may cause mechanical locking symptoms.
C. Radial
D. Horizontal: more common in older population

Medial meniscal tears: more common than lateral tears, the exception is in the setting of an acute ACL tear where lateral tears are more common. Degenerative tears in older patients usually occur in the posterior horn medial meniscus
Lateral meniscal tears: more common in acute ACL tear

Can you name the ligamentous structures that are responsible for knee stability?

Medial Collateral Ligament (MCL)
Lateral Collateral Ligament (LCL)

EXAMINATION

Anterior Cruciate Ligament (ACL)
Posterior Cruciate Ligament (PCL)
Popliteofibular Ligament / Posterior Lateral Corner (PLC)

Can you describe the function of MCL, LCL, PCL?

1. LCL: resists varus displacement
2. MCL: resists valgus angulation
3. PLC: resists posterolateral rotation of the tibia on the femur

Which is the most injured knee ligament, mechanism of injury and most common associated injuries?

MCL is the most commonly injured ligament of the knee
Mechanism of injury
Valgus and external rotation force to the lateral knee. Non-contact force results in milder sprains while direct blow usually causes complete disruption of MCL.
Rupture usually occurs at femoral insertion of ligament with proximal tears having greater healing rates
Associated conditions
1. ACL tears: comprise up to 95% of associated injuries
2. Meniscal tears: up to 5% of isolated MCL injuries are associated with meniscal tears

How can you assess the severity of MCL injury?

Classification of MCL Sprains
Grade 1
Mild severity
No loss of ligamentous integrity (stretch injury)
Minimal torn fibers
Grade II
Moderate severity
Incomplete tearing of MCL (partial tear)
Increased joint laxity
End point found at 30 degrees of flexion with valgus stress
Fibers remain apposed
Grade III
Severe
Complete disruption of ligament (complete tear)
Gross laxity, no end point with valgus stress at 30 degrees of knee flexion

How would you treat MCL injury?

Nonoperative:
Grade I: NSAIDs, rest, and physiotherapy.
Grades II and grade III: bracing, NSAIDs, rest and physiotherapy.

Operative
Ligament repair vs. reconstruction
Indications
1. Acute repair in grade III injuries.
2. In the setting of multi-ligament knee injury.
3. Continued instability despite nonoperative treatment.

Can you describe the anatomy and function(s) of the cruciate ligaments?

The cruciate are named anterior or posterior with regard to their positions of attachment on the tibial plateau.
A. ACL:
Tibial attachment: anterior intercondylar area of the tibial plateau.
Femoral attachment: the medial wall of the lateral femoral condyle.
B. PCL:
Tibial attachment: posterior intercondylar area of the tibial plateau.
Femoral attachment: lateral surface of the medial femoral condyle.

Function:
Anterior cruciate ligament: resists anterior translation of the tibia and internal tibia rotation especially at 90 degrees of flexion.
Posterior cruciate ligament: resists posterior tibial displacement especially at 90 degrees of flexion

Why is ACL injury more common in females?

ACL injury is more common in female athletes (4.5 :1 f/m ratio) due to:
1. Neuromuscular forces and control (more quadriceps dominant)
2. Landing biomechanics (conditioning and strength) play biggest role, females land in more extension, higher valgus moment
3. Smaller femoral notches
4. Genetic factors related to collagen production
5. Valgus leg alignment

How would you treat ACL injury?

Treatment
A. Nonoperative: physical therapy & lifestyle modifications
B. ACL reconstruction:
Indications:
1. Young and active patients (reduces incidence of meniscal or chondral injury).
2. Children (strongly consider operative as activity limitation is not realistic)
3. Older active patients (age >40 is not a contraindication if a high demand athlete)
4. ACL reconstruction failure
5. Associated injuries
MCL injury: allow MCL to heal (varus/valgus stability) and then perform ACL reconstruction because varus/valgus instability can jeopardize graft
Meniscal tear: perform meniscal repair at same time as ACL reconstruction as increased healing rate when repaired at the same time as ACL

What factors contribute to the stability of the patella-femoral joint?

The factors can be divided into the following:
A. Ligamentous Factors: medial patellar retinaculum.
B. Muscular Factors: oblique insertion of vastus medialis.
C. Bone stability: the prominent lateral condyle and deep trochlear groove of the distal femur.

Can you describe the anatomy and function of the medial capsulo-ligamentous complex of the knee?

It is composed of 3 layers which extend from the anterior midline to the posterior midline
It contains both static and dynamic stabilizers
Static stabilizers
Superficial MCL
Deep MCL and posterior oblique ligaments

Dynamic stabilizers
Consists of 5 attachments: vastus medialis, medial retinaculum, pes anserine muscle group
(Sartorius, semitendinosus, gracilis)
The function of the medial capsulo-ligamentous complex of the knee is to resist valgus and external forces at the knee.

SUMMARY OF EXAMINATION

Wash Your Hands
Ensure that you are seen by the examiners to wash your hands using alcohol gel provided.

Introduce, Explain, Expose and Inspect
Begin by introducing yourself, explain what you are going to do and check that this is OK with the patient and that he/she is not in any pain.
For knee examination the patient should be exposed to their underwear.

Inspect
Look for: symmetry, swelling, scars, muscle wasting.

Palpate
For any tenderness, temperature, extensor apparatus, knee effusion.

Movements
Active and passive flexion and extension.

Specific tests:
A. Ligaments
Collateral (varus and valgus stress test).
Cruciate (drawer/Lachman´s test).

B. Menisci
McMurray test

Closing
Thank the patient. Inform them that they may now get dressed or ensure they are adequately covered.
Present your findings to the examiner.

TOP TIPS

➕ Both Lachman's test for ACL injury and varus/valgus stress tests for collateral ligament injury should be performed with 20-30° knee flexion with the patient's heel on the couch.

➕ The predictor of success in meniscus repair is the distance from the tear to the peripheral meniscocapsular junction *(blood supply)*.

➕ MCL is the most commonly injured ligament of the knee.

1.20 | Foot and Ankle

Scenario

A 40 year old lady complains of a painful bunion on her forefoot. She has walking difficulty when wearing high-heeled shoes. She has had no previous injury to her feet.

The patient is comfortable, you have washed your hands, introduced yourself and explained what you are going to do. Please examine this lady's foot.

Describe how you would begin

Expose and Inspect: Adequate patient exposure, ideally with trousers/skirt off. First ask the patient to walk away a few steps, turn around and come back.

A. Standing position:
Inspect legs, ankles, feet, feet arches, and toes for scars, swelling, muscle wasting and any obvious deformity like intoeing, flat foot.
Ask the patient to walk on her tip-toes (plantar flexors).
Ask the patient to walk on her heels (dorsiflexors).
Ask the patient to stand on the outside edges of her feet.
Ask the patient to stand on the inside edges of her feet.

B. Sitting position:
Heel: exostosis, bursitis, old fracture.
Dorsum: dorsalis pedis pulse, exostosis, ganglion.
Big toe: hallux valgus, bunion, hallux rigidus.
Sole: callus, ulcers, verruca.

ᏦᎧ Inspection Findings

There is marked hallux valgus in the right foot with prominence of the first metatarsal head. There is also widening of the forefoot, bunion and medial rotation of the hallux.

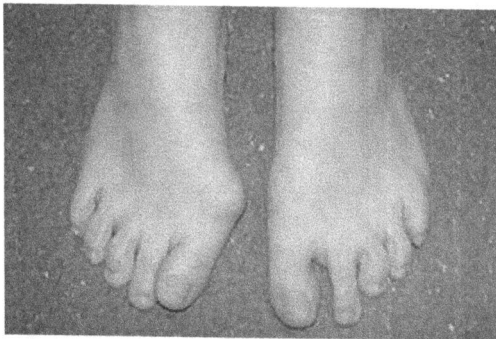

EXAMINATION

Having inspected what would you do next?

Next steps are feel, move and specific tests.

A. Feel (palpation): By palpation you are looking for the following (ask about pain before you palpate):
1. Pain: Heel (Sever's disease, exostosis, fasciitis, bursitis), forefoot, medial malleolus (tarsal tunnel syndrome), big toe.
2. Achilles tendon: palpate for defect, then palpate whilst the patient plantar-flexes against resistance.
3. Joint crepitations.
4. Temperature.

B. Move:
Ankle joint: hold the shin still and grip the whole heel. Move the foot, there should be plantar flexion (about 55°) and dorsiflexion (about 15°).
Subtalar joint: hold the ankle stable and grip the lower heel. Move the heel, there should be inversion (about 10°) and eversion (about 10°).
Forefoot (midtarsal and tarsometatarsal): hold the heel still and grip the forefoot, there should be inversion (15°), eversion (10°).
Metatarsophalangeal joints (MTPJ): check plantar and dorsal flexion.

C. Specific tests:

A. Tests for ankle stability:
There are three main ligaments around the ankle:
1. Lateral ligament from fibula to talus and calcaneus. Feel for it below the lateral malleolus. Test it by forcibly inverting the foot, if lax it will open up.
2. Medial (deltoid) ligament from the tibia to the talus, navicular, calcaneus and spring ligament. Feel for it below the medial malleolus. Test it by forcibly everting the foot; if lax it will open up.
3. The inferior tibiofibular ligament. Feel for it just above the joint line on the dorsal surface of the ankle between the fibula and tibia. Test for it by dorsiflexing the foot (will produce pain) and trying to move the talus laterally (will displace laterally if ligament is disrupted).

B. Tests for tenosynovitis:
Flexors/invertors: palpate along the tendons behind the medial malleolus. Milk out synovial fluid from the tendon by running fingers proximally along them.
Tibialis posterior: plantarflexion and eversion of the foot will precipitate pain just posterior to the medial malleolus.
Peroneal tendons: plantarflexion and inversion of the foot will precipitate pain behind the lateral malleolus. Ask the patient to evert against resistance and feel for snapping of thickened peroneal tendons.

C. Thompson's test: position the patient prone with their feet off the edge of the couch. Squeezing the calf should cause plantar flexion of the ankle. If not, this is pathognomonic of a ruptured Achilles tendon.

D. Tinel's tarsal tunnel test: Percuss the posterior tibial nerve as it runs through the tarsal tunnel.
This is located posterior to the medial malleolus. Reproduction of the symptoms suggests tarsal tunnel syndrome.

👓 Findings

The patient has pain over the head of the first metatarsal bone (bunion). Normal range of motion at all joints including first metatarsophalangeal joint. Foot X-ray shows abnormal first MPJ angle and no osteoarthritis changes in the MTPJ.

Foot x – ray

EXAMINATION

Given the history and examination findings this is likely to be hallux valgus of the right foot.

How would you manage this patient?

A. Nonoperative:
Wide shoes, padding to protect bunions, anterior platform support to relieve metatarsalgia.
B. Operative:
a) Mild/moderate deformity: Distal soft tissue realignment with distal osteotomy of first metatarsal (e.g. Mitchell's osteotomy).
b) Severe deformity: shaft osteotomy or proximal osteotomy.

Can you describe the component(s) of hallux valgus deformity?

Hallux valgus is a complex deformity of the first ray and consists of one or a combination of the following deformities:
1. Valgus deviation of the phalanx promotes varus position of metatarsal bone.
2. The metatarsal head displaces medially, leaving the sesamoid complex laterally translated relative to the metatarsal head.
3. Sesamoids remain within the respective head of the flexor hallucis brevis tendon and are attached to the base of the proximal phalanx which leads to valgus deviation of the phalanx. This lateral displacement can lead to transfer metatarsalgia due to a shift in weight bearing.
4. Medial MTPJ capsule becomes stretched and attenuated while the lateral capsule becomes contracted.
5. Adductor tendon becomes a deforming force, inserts on fibular sesamoid and lateral aspect of proximal phalanx.

6. Plantar and lateral migration of the abductor hallucis causes muscle to plantar flex and pronate phalanx.

What is the first metatarsophalangeal angle?

First metatarsophalangeal angle is formed by a line drawn in plain X-ray through the longitudinal axis of the first metatarsal with that drawn through the longitudinal axis of the first proximal phalanx. A normal angle is less than 15°.

Name the Associated conditions with hallux valgus?

Associated conditions:
1. Hammer toe deformity.
2. Callosities.
3. Hallux rigidus.

What are the possible complications following surgical treatment?

Complications:
1. Recurrence
2. Avascular necrosis of metatarsal head
3. Dorsal malunion with transfer metatarsalgia
4. Hallux Varus
5. Cock-up toe deformity
6. Neuropraxia: Painful incisional neuromas after bunion surgery frequently involve the medial branch of the dorsal cutaneous nerve – a terminal branch of the superficial peroneal nerve.

Can you describe hammer toe deformity?

Hammer deformity characterized by: flexion of the PIP joint, extension deformity at DIP. Deformity can be rigid or flexible.

Can you describe treatment of hammer toe deformity?

A. Nonoperative:
Shoes with high toe boxes, foam or silicone gel sleeves
B. Operative:
1. Flexor tendon (FDL) to extensor tendon transfer.
   Indications
   Flexible deformity that has failed nonoperative management
2. Resection arthroplasty +/ – tenotomy and tendon transfers
   Indications
   Rigid deformity that has failed nonoperative management

Can you describe the nerve supply of the foot?

A. Branches of the Tibial nerve:
1. Medial calcaneal nerve innervates plantar medial heel.
2. Medial plantar nerve innervates abductor hallucis, FHB, FDB, lumbricals to 2nd and 3rd toes.
3. Lateral plantar nerve innervates (everything else), adductor hallucis, quadratus plantae, all interossei muscles, lateral two lumbricals, abductor digiti minimus (via Baxter's nerve – the first branch of LPN).
B. Sural Nerve:
Provides dorsal sensory in 4th web space
C. Deep peroneal Nerve:

Innervates EDB, and EHB in foot. Provides sensation to the first dorsal webspace.
D. Superficial Peroneal Nerve:
Provides sensation to the dorsum of the foot (with the exception of the first web space, which is innervated by the deep peroneal nerve).
E. Saphenous Nerve:
Supplies sensation to medial side of foot.

Can you describe the different parts of the foot, joints and movements that is/are produced by each?

1. **Hindfoot**
   Consists of articulation between talus and calcaneus.
   Joints:
   A. Subtalar joint:
   It has 3 facets: posterior facet, middle facet which is located medially and sits on the sustentaculum of the calcaneus, anterior facet which is continuous with the talonavicular joint.
   Motion:
   inversion/eversion.
   B. Transverse tarsal joint (Chopart joint):
   Consists of two components: talonavicular joint and calcaneocuboid joint.
   Motion:
   Inversion of subtalar joint locks the transverse tarsal joint which allows for a stable hindfoot/midfoot for toe-off. Eversion of subtalar joint unlocks the transverse tarsal joint which allows for supple foot to accommodate ground just after heel strike.
2. **Midfoot**
   Starts at the articulation between the navicular and cuneiforms.
   Joints:
   A. Naviculocuneiform and intercuneiform joints.
   B. Tarsometatarsal joint (Lisfranc joint): divided into three columns. Medial column is composed of first metatarsal, medial cuneiform and navicular. Middle column is composed of second and third metatarsals, middle cuneiform and lateral cuneiform, lateral column is composed of fourth, fifth metatarsals and cuboid.
   Motion:
   Lateral column is the most mobile, allows for flexibility when walking on uneven ground.
   middle column is the least mobile, allows for rigidity during push-off.
   medial column carries most of the load while standing.
3. **Forefoot**
   Extends from tarsal-metatarsal joint to tips of toes. Bones consists of: phalanges and metatarsals.
   Joints:
   metarsalphalangeal joints
   proximal interphalangeal joints
   distal interphalangeal joints
   Motion:
   Flexion/extension

What are the different phases of normal gait?

One gait cycle is measured from heel-strike to heel-strike. It consists of:
1. **Stance phase**
   Period of time when the foot is on the ground. About 60% of one gait cycle is spent in stance phase.
   During stance phase, the leg accepts body weight and provides single limb support.

2. Swing phase
Period of time when the foot is off the ground moving forward. About 40% of one gait cycle is spent In Swing phase. The foot swings forward (to become the leading foot again) and the contralateral foot supports the body.

What different types of gait do you know of?

1. Antalgic: decreased stance and increased swing phase on the affected leg (due to pain).
2. Cerebellar: broad based gait.
3. High stepping: Due to foot drop (commonly due to peroneal nerve damage).
4. Parkinsonian: shuffling gait.
5. Spastic: jerky and scissoring.
6. Trendelenberg: the patient lurches over the side of the bad hip to compensate for abductor weakness.

SUMMARY OF EXAMINATION

Wash Your Hands
Ensure that you are seen by the examiners to wash your hands using alcohol gel provided.

Introduce, Explain, Expose and Inspect
Begin by introducing yourself, explain what you are going to do and check that this is OK with the patient and that he/she is not in any pain.
For ankle and foot examination the patient should be ideally with trousers/ skirt off.

Look
Inspect both at standing (from the front, back and sides) and in sitting position and observe for any scars, swelling, symmetry, deformity and muscle wasting.

Feel
Palpate systematically for any tenderness over the bony structures and soft tissue.

Move
Dorsiflexion/plantar flexion (ankle joint), inversion/eversion (subtalar joint), flexion and extension (toes).

Specific tests
Tests for ankle stability
Tests for tenosynovitis
Thompson´s test
Tinel´s tarsal tunnel syndrome

Closing
Thank the patient. Inform them that they may now get dressed or ensure they are adequately covered.
Present your findings to the examiner.

EXAMINATION

TOP TIPS

➕ First ask the patient to walk away and assess the pattern of gait before starting examination.

➕ Remember to compare each side, starting with good side first.

➕ Complete the examination by examining the distal neurovascular status.

EXAMINATION

1.21 | Cranial Nerve

Scenario

A 67-year-old long-term smoker presents with ptosis of the left eye, intermittent haemoptysis and weight loss. On examination he has crepitations of the left lung base and ptosis of the left eye. A CXR is performed which reveals an apical lung tumour on the left side.

"The patient is comfortable, you have washed your hands, introduced yourself and explained what you are going to do. Please examine…"

Describe how you would begin

Ensure adequate exposure of the patient, sit an arms length away and directly opposite the patient .

Inspection Findings

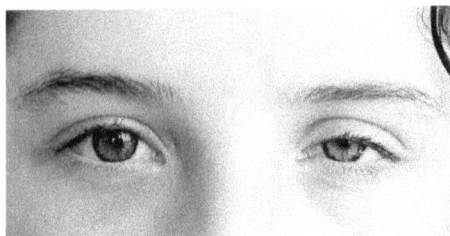

Figure 1

Describe what you see on inspection

On inspection, the right eye appears normal, but in contrast, on the left side, the eyelid is drooping (ptosis) and the left pupil is smaller than on the right side. (Figure 1)

Having inspected what would you do next?

Examine the cranial nerves involved and eye movements. Perform visual acuity tests..
Cranial Nerve II – Optic Nerve:
- Start assessing cranial nerve II by testing for visual acuity, using a Snellen Chart.
- Ask the patient to look directly ahead and shine the pen torch into one pupil, followed by the other. Look for both a direct and consensual reflex. Also test for an afferent pupillary nerve defect using the 'swinging light test' between the pupils
- Assess the fundus in each eye with an ophthalmoscope
- Ask the patient to look straight over your shoulder at your fist and then at your finger in front of their face to assess accommodation (pupillary constriction and convergence on near target)
- Test for visual field defects, by asking the patient to look at a fixed point and while sitting opposite them, test the four quadrants (Figure 2) – it is important to test one eye at a time (cover the eye that is not being tested) and compare to your own.
- Assess colour vision using Ishihara plates – This is not usually covered in the

EXAMINATION

examination station.

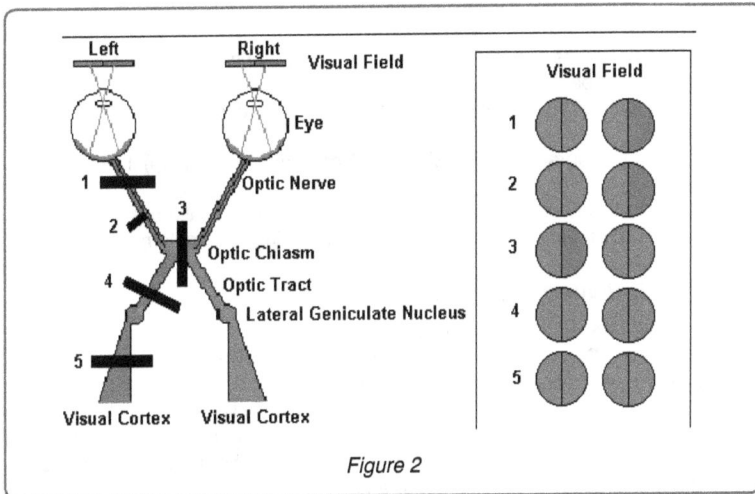

Figure 2

Cranial Nerve III – Occulomotor Nerve, Cranial Nerve IV – Trochlear Nerve, Cranial Nerve VI – Abducens Nerve:
Ask the patient to follow your finger when making an 'H' sign, noting any restriction of movement, diplopia or pain. CN III forms the efferent component of the pupillary light response, but is usually assessed as part of the examination of CN II. Access the pupillary response to evaluate the integrity of the third nerve.

Differential diagnosis

- Third nerve palsy (occulomotor) – ptosis, dilated, poorly reactive pupil, reduced occular movements in directions.
  - Surgical – Due to intracranial lesions or space occupying lesions.
  - Medical – 'Pupil sparing' third nerve palsy, usually diabetic related
  - Horner's Syndrome – Interruption of the sympathetic pathway to the eye, with, impairment of Muller's muscle, leading to partial ptosis, miosis and anhidrosis (lack of sweating on the affected side). It may be impaired at any part along its length in the head, neck, chest or paraspinally.
  - Myasthenia Gravis – Autoimmune condition of the neuromuscular junction (NMJ) causing fatigable ptosis and third nerve signs (usually bilateral).
  - Weber's Syndrome – Ipsilateral third nerve palsy with contralateral hemiparesis associated with
- Fourth Nerve Palsy (Trochlear) – Vertical diplopia in the absence of ptosis. Commonly congenital, less often traumatic. Intracranial masses rarely present with an isolated IVth nerve palsy.
- Sixth Nerve Palsy (Abducens) – Inability to abduct the affected eye. Can be associated with any cause of raised intra cranial pressure and nasopharyngeal tumours or basal skull fractures.

EXAMINATION

How will you manage the patient?

Manage according to ATLS Principles if traumatic head injury suspected Investigations should include:

- Random Blood Glucose – In patients over 50 years, with risk factors who have a pupil sparing third nerve palsy
- CXR – if Horner's syndrome suspected from apical lung cancer
- Neuroimaging
  - CT Cerebral Angiogram or MRA (Magnetic Resonance Angiogram) if aneurysm suspected
  - CT Head if not isolated third nerve palsy and other intracranial mass suspected
- CSF Analysis – CSF sample testing if associated meningitic symptoms are present

Differences between similar conditions

- Horner's Syndrome: Miosis, anhydrosis, partial ptosis
- Third nerve palsy: Complete ptosis, pupillary dilatation (in surgical third nerve palsy), paralysis of accommodation, down and out deviation,
- Fourth Nerve Palsy: Paralysis of the superior oblique muscle, causing the eye to look down with vertical diplopia. Has a long course, often damaged in traumatic brain injury.
- Sixth Nerve Palsy: Paralysis of the lateral rectus muscle. The patient is unable to abduct the eye (look laterally), but able to adduct fully.

Follow-on questions

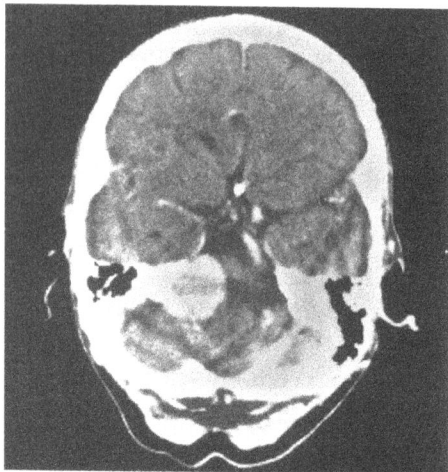

Describe this CT scan. What are your differentials and which nerve is likely to be affected and why?

This is an axial CT scan with contrast that demonstrates a mass lesion in the cerebellopontine angle. Differential diagnoses would include vestibular schwannoma and meningioma. Indicating a right acoustic neuroma. The sixth nerve is usually affected in these lesions as it arises from the pontomedullary junction.

EXAMINATION

What is the difference between medical and surgical third nerve palsy?

If the pupil is spared it is sometimes referred to as a 'medical' third nerve palsy, whereas if it is fixed and dilated it is a 'surgical' third nerve palsy.

Does the abducens nerve consist of motor and sensory components?

No the abducens nerve is purely motor to innervate the lateral rectus muscle, which abducts the eye.

What is the function of the superior oblique muscle and what nerve supplies it?

The superior oblique muscle depresses, abducts and medially rotates the eyeball. It is supplied by the trochlear nerve (Cranial Nerve IV).

SUMMARY OF EXAMINATION

Wash Your Hands
Ensure that you are seen by the examiners to wash your hands using alcohol gel provided.

Introduce, Explain, Expose and Inspect
Begin by introducing yourself, explain what you are going to do and check that this is ok with the patient and that he/she is not in any pain.
For cranial nerve eye examinations, ensure that you are sat opposite and an arm's distance from the patient.

Inspect
Inspect for eye signs, note the position and size of the pupil. Note any associated features such as anhydrosis.

Assessment of cranial nerves II, III, IV and VI
Test for each of the cranial nerves in turn.
Position the patient appropriately, assessing acuity, pupillary response, fundoscopy, accommodation and visual fields.
Test cranial nerves III, IV and VI by asking the patient to follow the 'H' shape with their eyes and assessing for restricted movement and for diplopia.
Auscultate the lungs if Horner's Syndrome is likely.

Closing
Thank the patient. Inform them that they may now get dressed or ensure they are adequately covered.
Present your findings to the examiner.

Wash Your Hands
Ensure that you are seen by the examiners to wash your hands using alcohol gel provided.

EXAMINATION

TOP TIPS

➕ The examiners are looking for a fluent examination, so practice using a variety of approaches

➕ Have an idea of the path of the cranial nerves, particularly III, IV and IV in mind so interpreting neuroimaging or linking specific nerve involvements to the site of injury on the skull or the location of intra cranial masses maybe made easier

➕ Don't forget to mention that a full neurovascular examination maybe warranted and if any of the above nerves are impaired, a full cranial nerve examination should also be conducted.

1.22 | Upper Limb Neurology

Station Name

Upper Limb Peripheral Nerves – Ulnar Nerve (Cubital Tunnel Compression)

> ### Scenario
>
> A 56-year-old lady presents with a 12-week history of right elbow tenderness, initially intermittent and now constant. She has known osteoarthritis, but is otherwise well. She reports tingling in the little finger and the ulnar half of the ring finger on the right hand. She has also noticed a loss of function of the right hand, with clawing of the little and ring fingers and loss of grip strength on the right side.
>
> "The patient is comfortable; you have washed you hands, introduced yourself and explained what you are going to do. Please examine…"

Describe how you would begin

Expose the patient adequately, allowing full range of movement at the elbow and ensuring the joint above and below are exposed. Ask the patient regarding any tenderness over the right elbow

👓 Inspection Findings

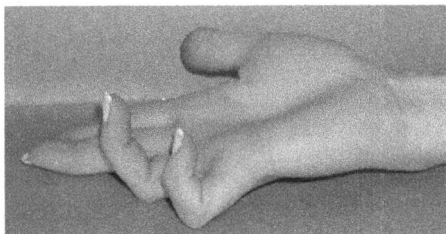

Figure 1: Ulnar Claw Hand

Describe what you see on inspection

The elbow position is held in a valgus deformity. The right hand is held in a 'claw-like' position with extension at the MCPJ and flexion of the DIPJ/PIPJ in the ring and little finger and the little finger is abducted (Wartenburg's sign). Additionally, there is some wasting of the intrinsic muscles of the hand and the hypothenar eminence.

Having inspected what would you do next?

The hand is held in the position shown above.
Sensation: There is reduced sensation to light touch over the little and ulnar half of the ring finger on the right hand, the hypothenar eminence and the dorsum of the hand, in the distribution shown below.
Movements: The patient is unable to abduct the fingers or adduct the fingers against resistance, as the ulnar nerve supplies the intrinsic muscles of the hand.
Palpation & Special tests: Over the medial epicondyle causes pain. On tapping over the

EXAMINATION

medial epicondyle, paraesthesia is felt in the hand within the ulnar nerve distribution (ulnar tap test).

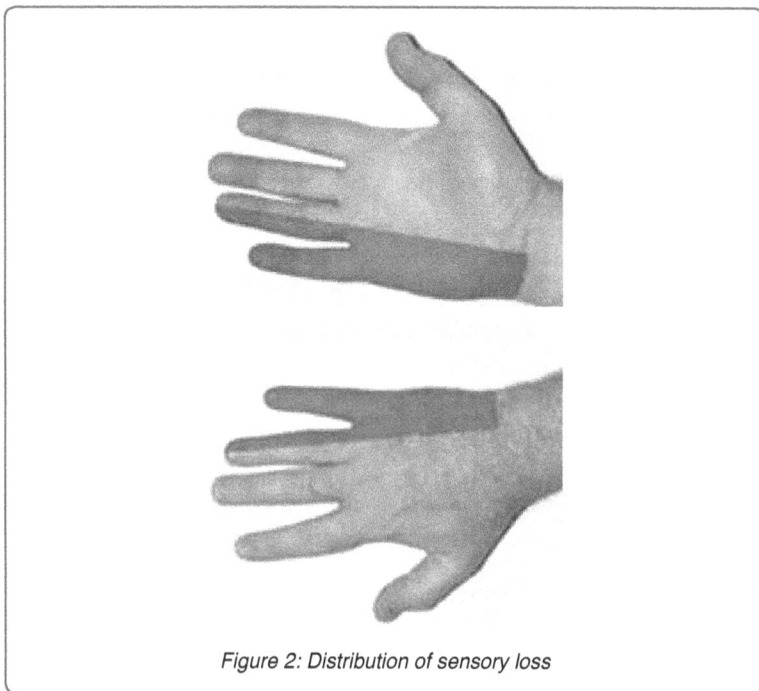

Figure 2: Distribution of sensory loss

Froment's Sign:
Is tested by asking the patient to hold a piece of paper between the thumb and index finger (with the thumb adducted fully). In ulnar nerve palsy, failure of contraction of adductor pollicis usually results in contraction of flexor pollicis longus (supplied by the anterior interosseus nerve) instead and therefore thumb flexion (at the IP joint) occurs to keep hold of the paper.

Differential diagnosis

- Damage to Ulnar Nerve: At the wrist due to compression in Guyon's canal or in the hand due to deep motor branch compression against the pisiform and hamate – usually in those persons using vibrating tools.
- Inflammation of the ulnar nerve itself called ulnar nerve nerititis or contusion or nearby structures, such as medial epicondyle leading to medial epicondylitis or 'Golfer's Elbow'may cause symptoms.
- Others include lower trunk brachial plexus injury, brachial neuritis, thoracic outlet syndrome, or C8/T1 nerve root compression.
- Cubitus valgus, a deformity at the elbow associated with supracondylar fractures in childhood may also cause cubital tunnel syndrome.

How will you manage the patient?

Investigations
- Biochemistry - Random glucose to test for diabetes mellitus.
Imaging:
- USS – to diagnose cubital tunnel and the cause, site and diameter of the lesion.

- Radiographs –of the elbow and wrist to rule out 'double crush syndrome', caused by reduced axoplasmic flow in patients with suspected traumatic injury,
- Nerve conduction studies/Electromyography (NCS/EMG) – Can confirm a diagnosis of cubital tunnel syndrome both absolute and relative reduction in conduction velocity compared to a normal section of the ulnar nerve. It may also differentiate nerve root pathology and the site of compression along the ulnar nerve for example at the thoracic outlet, cubital tunnel or Guyon's Canal.
- MRI – Can be useful to rule out injuries to the brachial plexus or cervical root pathology

Management
Conservative:
Physiotherapy, nocturnal splinting and occupational therapy
Medical:
Analgesia Non Steroidal Anti-inflammatory Drugs and vitamin B6/B12 supplementation
Surgical:
Offered for patients with persistent paraesthesia, weakness or progressive disease.
- Surgical decompression – for cases of cubital tunnel syndrome, the nerve can be freed from the cubital tunnel and transposed anteriorly
- Medial epicondylectomy – in the event of compression at the level of the medial epicondyle. Nerve can also be transposed.

Differences between similar conditions

- How to differentiate ulnar nerve palsy vs. a C8 lesion: A C8 lesion is accompanied by weakness of wrist extension.
- How to differentiate ulnar nerve palsy vs. a T1 lesion: Loss of sensation over the T1 dermatome, with weakness of abductor pollicis brevis

Follow on questions

What is the path of the ulnar nerve?

The ulnar nerve pierces the intermuscular septum at level of mid-humerus and runs with triceps, then behind the medial epicondyle and into the forearm, running between the two heads of flexor carpi ulnaris. Above the wrist, it gives off the dorsal cutaneous branch, then passes into Guyon's canal, superficial to flexor retinaculum, with the ulnar artery

What movements test the ulnar nerve specifically?

- Ulnar wrist flexion flexor carpi ulnaris
- Palmar and dorsal interossei – PAD and DAB
  Palmar interossi = Adduct
  Dorsal interossei – Abduct
- Flexion of the MCPJ
- Abduction of the little finger (abductor digiti minimi)

What are the cord values of the ulnar nerve and what muscles does it supply?

The cord values for the ulnar nerve are C8 and T1, from the medial cord of the brachial plexus.. The ulnar nerve supplies the muscles flexor carpi ulnaris and ulna half of flexor digitorum profundus of the 4th and 5th fingers and the interossei.

The patient holds the little finger in abduction, what is this sign called and why does it occur?

Wartenburg's sign and is due to the unopposed action of abductor digiti minimi on the little finger.

EXAMINATION

What is the ulnar paradox?

This is to do with the level of the lesion affecting the ulnar nerve. A high ulnar lesion causes less clawing of the hand. A low ulnar lesion causes more clawing of the hand. This is because in low ulnar lesions, flexor digitorum profundus, which supplies the little and ulnar half of the ring finger is intact, making the clawing of the hand worse. So paradoxically a lower ulnar nerve lesion produces a worse claw hand.

SUMMARY OF EXAMINATION

Wash Your Hands: Ensure that you are seen by the examiners to wash your hands using alcohol gel provided.

Introduce, Explain, Expose and Inspect
Begin by introducing yourself, explain what you are going to do and check that this is ok with the patient and that he/she is not in any pain.
To examine the cubital tunnel, expose the patients elbow and ideally the joint above and below.

Inspect
Inspect for scars, deformity and any erythema

Palpate
The patient is examined systematically, by inspection of the elbow joint, in particular the medial epicondyle. The cubital tunnel is palpated and any exacerbation of symptoms noted. The ulnar tap test or Tinel's sign at the elbow is performed. Sensation in the ulnar nerve distribution and power are tested prior to commencing special tests such as Froment's Sign.

Froment's Test:
To perform the test, a patient is asked to hold an object, usually a flat object such as a piece of paper, between their thumb and index finger (pinch grip). The examiner then attempts to pull the object out of the subject's hands.
• A normal individual will be able to maintain a hold on the object without difficulty.
• However, with ulnar nerve palsy, the patient will experience difficulty maintaining a hold and will compensate by flexing the FPL (flexor pollicis longus) of the thumb to maintain grip pressure causing a pinching effect.
• Clinically, this compensation manifests as flexion of the IP joint of the thumb (rather than adduction, as would occur with correct use of the adductor pollicis).

Upper Limb Motor Function
'I'm now going to test the nerves in your arms.'
Compare both limbs

Inspect
'Are you right or left handed?'
Look at skin, muscles and look for wasting and fasciculations.
Pronator drift – arms outstretched, palms facing up, eyes closed. Pronation=weakness on that side

Tone
Isolate the limb. Hold the joint above and move the limb. Compare sides.
Power

Deltoid (C5,6) –ask patient to raise arm up like a chicken wing, hold shoulder. 'Don't let me move your arm'.
Biceps (C5,6) –ask patient to raise forearms up like a boxer, hold elbow. 'Stop me from pushing, stop me from pulling'.
Wrist (C7,8)– hold wrist 'stop me from pushing up and pushing down on outstretched fingers'/'grip my fingers'
Fingers (C8,T1) – 'spread your fingers apart and stop me from trying to close them.'

Reflexes

Ask patient to relax their arms and rest them in their lap.
Biceps tendon (C5) – finger on tendon and hit finger using tendon hammer. Compare sides.
Triceps tendon (C7) – hold arm up slightly and hit behind elbow
Supinator tendon (C6) – radial aspect 10cm above wrist joint

Sensation

Pain (Spinothalamic)
Use neurotip. 'I'm going to press this onto your arm. I'd like you to close your eyes and say 'Yes' when you can feel it.'
Test dermatomes. Compare both arms. 'Was it the same feeling on both sides?'
Remember to dispose of neurotip after use.
Arm Dermatomes: See map at end of sheet. From outside shoulder: C5, C6, C7(middle finger), C8, T1, T2

Proprioception (Dorsal Column)
'I'd like you to close your eyes and tell me whether your finger is up or down?'
Hold patient's terminal phalanx between thumb and forefinger on either side while immobilising the proximal phalanx with other hand.

Vibration (Dorsal Column)
With patient's eyes closed place tuning fork on little finger or wrist. 'Can you feel that? Now tell me when it stops.'

Light touch (Spinothalamic)
Use cotton wool. 'I'm going to press this onto your arm. I'd like you to say 'Yes' when you can feel it.'
Test dermatomes moving up from little finger and then thumb sides. 'Was it the same feeling on both sides?']

Coordination

Ask patient to pretend to play the piano
Ask patient to touch their nose and then touch your finger, move finger around and keep at patient's maximum reach.
Ask patient to rapidly pronate and supinate left hand onto dorsum of right hand. Then swap hands. (Dysdiadochokinesis)

TOP TIPS

➕ Ensure that you understand the tests and movements in the hand for each specific nerve – radial, median and ulnar.

➕ Have an efficient way of testing the sensation for each of the nerves above quickly

EXAMINATION

1.23 | Lower Limb Neurology

Scenario

A 35-year-old man is brought in after a road traffic accident. You attend the A&E trauma call. He is stable after the primary survey, however on the secondary survey radiographs reveal that he has a fracture at the neck of the left fibula. On examination he is unable to dorsiflex the foot and has loss of sensation over the lower lateral leg and dorsum of the foot.

The patient is comfortable, you have washed your hands, introduced yourself and explained what you are going to do. Given the history above, please examine the lower limb.

EXAMINATION

Describe how you would begin

- Observe the area around the patient looking for walking aids and check the soles of shoes for asymmetrical wear. Observe the lower limb from all sides, including posteriorly.
- Look for asymmetry, breeching of or compromised skin over the fracture site and bruising over the proximal fibula.

Inspection Findings

On inspection you find bruising and swelling over the proximal aspect of the fibula on the left leg. The skin is intact, but there is an area of compromised skin over the head of the fibula. There is no obvious deformity of the lower limb.

Having inspected what would you do next?

Move:
- Ask the patient to walk towards and away from you, inspecting the gait ('high stepping' or 'foot-slapping')
- Check for foot drop asking the patient to walk 'heel to toes'
- Test plantar flexion of the foot – S1/2 by asking the patient to stand on their tiptoes
- Test for dorsiflexion of the foot – L4/5 by asking the patient to stand on their heels
- Assess for weakness of extensor hallucis longus
- Test inversion and eversion of the foot (inversion spared with common peroneal nerve palsy)

Sensation:
- Test for sensation over the lower lateral leg and dorsum of the foot – superficial peroneal nerve, reduced in foot drop
- Test for sensation over the first web space – Deep peroneal nerve, reduced in foot drop
- Test for sensation over the medial aspect of the foot – saphenous nerve, should be intact
- Test for sensation over the lateral aspect of the foot – sural nerve, should be intact

Summary:

		Motor	Sensory
1	Deep Peroneal Nerve	Loss of ant.tibialis and ankle dorsiflexion (L4/5)	Loss of sensation first webspace
2	Superficial Peroneal Nerve	loss of peroneus longus/brevis and foot eversion (L5/S1)	Loss of sensation over lateral distal leg
3	Common Peroneal Nerve	Includes motor and sensory loss from both deep (1) and superficial (2) peroneal nerves	
4	Radiculopathy of L4/5	Includes motor loss from both deep (1) and superficial (2) peroneal Nerves. In addition to loss of tibialis posterior and foot inversion (L4/5).	Sensory loss is dermatomal over L4/5.
5	Sciatic Nerve (Main Trunk)	Loss of ankle dorsiflexion, foot eversion, foot inversion, knee flexion (biceps femoris – L5/S1/S2) and plantarflexion (Gastrocnemius-S1/S2)	Loss of sensation over lateral leg and whole of foot.

Reflexes:
Increased in upper motor neurone lesions and decreased in lower motor neurone lesions. Reflexes of lower limb include knee (L3/4) and ankle (S1).

Differential diagnosis

- Nerve Root Compression: L4 or L5 nerve root compression,
- Sciatic Nerve Injury or compression
- Common peroneal nerve palsy (trauma/ compression from POP cast)
- Medical: Peripheral neuropathies (including diabetes/alcohol induced neuropathy)
- Hyper flexion of the knee, fractures to distal femur or dislocation of knee

How will you manage the patient?

Relevant Investigations:
- Blood tests (FBC, U&E, Random glucose, HbA1C, B12 and folate) – If suspect malignancy / peripheral neuropathy
- Imaging
  - Peripheral lesions: MRI Lumbar spine/lumbosacral plexus; Central Lesions: MRI brain to look for parasagittal lesions
  - Plain films – to access bony damage and direct avulsion or fractures leading to compartment syndrome
- Neurophysiology – NCS/EMG
- Invasive – CSF sampling if infiltrative malignancy suspected

Differences between similar conditions

Compartment syndrome – may also lead to foot drop
Lumbosacral plexopathy – Involving the nerve root values of the common peroneal nerve (L4-S1)
Intra-operative injury should be considered if foot drop noted after total knee replacement

What is the cutaneous sensation of the deep and superficial peroneal nerves?

The superficial peroneal nerve innervates the anterolateral/distal leg and dorsum of the

EXAMINATION

foot. The deep peroneal nerve innervates the skin of the 1st dorsal web space of the foot (between the first and second toes).

What are the different kinds of nerve damage?

Seddon Classification
Neuropraxia – Demyelination, with conduction block
Axonotemesis – Disruption of the nerve fibres, endoneurium intact
Neurotemesis – Three types: 1. Endoneurium disrupted/perineurium intact; 2. Perineurium interrupted, epineurium intact; 3. Nerve severed, complete disruption of the epineurium.

How does the prognosis differ with each?

Neuropraxia usually fully recovers. Axonotemesis with the endoneurium intact allows the nerve to regenerate. Neurotemesis results in a poor prognosis for regeneration, as both the perineurium and endoneurium are injured.

What muscles does the common peroneal nerve innervate?

The common peroneal nerve directly innervates the short head of the biceps femoris. The remainder of the muscles innervated by the nerve are via its branches, the superficial peroneal nerve and the deep peroneal nerve. The superficial peroneal nerve supplies muscles in the lateral compartment of the lower leg, peroneus longus and brevis, which are primarily evertors of the foot. The deep peroneal nerve supplies the anterior compartment of the nerve, innervating the tibialis anterior, extensor hallucis longus/brevis and extensor digitorum longus/brevis.

From which nerve is the common peroneal a continuation of? What are the nerve root values for this nerve?

The common peroneal nerve is a continuation of the sciatic nerve, the root values of which are L4, L5, S1, S2, and S3.

SUMMARY OF EXAMINATION

Motor

Inspect

Look at skin, muscles and look for wasting and fasciculations.

Tone

Shake/roll leg. Let leg go floppy and drop from the knee.

Test clonus by revolving ankle and then rapidly dorsiflex to elicit beats. (Gastronemius muscle, >5 beats pathological)

Power

Hip (L1,2) – 'I'd like you to raise your left leg off he bed. And stop me from moving it.' Compare sides.

Knee (L3,4,5) – 'I'd like you to bend your knees. And stop me from moving them.

Ankle (L4,S1,2) – 'I'd like you to flex your ankle up towards you. And stop me from moving it.'

Toe (L5) – 'I'd like you to move your big toes towards you. And stop me from moving it.'

Reflexes

Knee (L3, L4)– Place hand underneath knees to take some of the weight. Use tendon hammer to elicit reflex.

Ankle (L5, S1) – relax by slightly flexing knee and slightly dorsiflexing ankle. Reinforce if necessary by asking patient to grasp and pull hands.

Plantar reflex (L5, S1) – Run finger along the lateral border of the sole of the foot from the heel to the toe. Normally produces plantar flexion of toes. In UMN lesion causes dorsiflexion – Babinski's sign.

Sensation

Pain (Spinothalamic)

Use neurotip. . 'I'm going to press this onto your leg. I'd like you to close your eyes and say 'Yes' when you can feel it.'

Compare legs. 'Was it the same on both sides?'

Proprioception (Dorsal Column)

With patient's eyes closed move big toe up and down. 'Tell me whether I'm moving your toe up or down.' Hold sides of toe between finger and immobilise foot.

Vibration (Dorsal Column)

Use tuning fork on medial maleolus. 'Say 'Yes' when you can feel the tuning fork. Now tell me when it stops.'

Light touch (Spinothalamic)

Use cotton wool. 'I'm going to press this onto your leg. I'd like you to say 'Yes' when you can feel it.'

Test dermatomes moving up from big toe and then little toe sides. 'Was it the same feeling on both sides?']

Coordination

'I'd like you to touch your left knee with your right heel. Now run your heel down your leg to your foot and do this as quickly as you can.' Then other leg.

Gait - Ask the patient to walk if appropriate.

1.24 | Breast

Scenario

A 43-year-old lady presents with a lump in the upper outer quadrant of the right breast. She is Gravida 2 Para 2 and is not currently breast-feeding. She is uncertain how long the lump has been present for. She has no nipple discharge or skin retraction over the breast lump. This lady previously underwent a mastectomy of the left breast with immediate reconstruction. There is no history of recent unintentional weight loss, but she has recently developed back pain over the thoracic vertebrae.

Describe how you would begin

Expose and Inspect: For breast examination the patient should be exposed from the waist up.
Observe the patient from the end of the best for shortness of breath, ask for a chaperone.
Patient Sitting:
- Ask the patient to sit facing you and observe for any obvious swelling, nipple discharge, skin retraction or previous scars (DIEP/ TRAM flaps produce a horizontal scar over the lower suprapubic area, LD flaps produce scars across the back, usually inferior to the scapula).
- Look for any evidence of radiotherapy tattooing or scars or lymphedema.
- Ask the patient to place their hands on their hips and push inwards to contract the pectoralis muscle to exaggerate any overlying breast lumps.
- Ask the patient to put their hands on their head to observe for any obvious lymphadenopathy or scars in the axillae.
- *Observe around the bed for any prosthetic bras, which the patient may have with them.*

> ### ⌢〰 Inspection Findings
>
>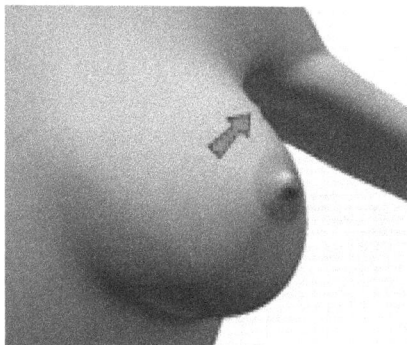

Describe the what you see on inspection

On contraction of the pectoralis muscle when sitting, this lady has a prominent lump in the right breast.

On inspection the lump appears to be in the right upper outer quadrant

On the left side, the nipple is absent; there is a scar over the left breast and at the back of the patient over the inferior boarder of the left scapula.

Having inspected what would you do next?

Palpate
Breast Lump:
Palpate the four quadrants of the examined breast; palpation of the upper outer quadrant should include the 'tail' of the pectoralis major muscle (the Tail of Spence).
Palpate the nipple-areolar complex.
If there is a palpable lump assess the lump for fluctuance, size, shape, mobility/tethering and any pain. Ask the patient to contract and access if the lump is adherent to the underlying muscle.

Lymph Nodes:
Palpate the cervical and axillary lymph nodes on both sides, accessing for enlarged nodes, consistency and nodularity.

At the end of the examination:
Liver:
Palpate for an enlarged liver, accessing for any nodularity, which may indicate liver metastasis.

Spine:
Tap down the patient's spine, accessing for any pain that may suggest spinal metastasis.

Respiratory:
Listen to the lung bases for evidence of pulmonary metastasis

Check for winging of the scapula (long thoracic nerve damage, C5, 6,7).

Findings

There is a 3 x 2 cm palpable lump in the upper outer quadrant of the right breast. There is no associated skin changes, discharge or scars over the right breast. The lump is firm and fixed to the underlying pectoralis muscle. There is a palpable lymph node in the apex of the right axillae. There is evidence of a previous mastectomy, with latissimus dorsi reconstruction on the left side. There is tenderness over the T8/T9 thoracic vertebrae on palpation.

What is your differential diagnosis?

Neoplasm of the breast – benign fibroadeoma or malignant – lobular or ductal cell carcinoma.
Inflammatory differentials include an abscess of the breast.

How would you manage this patient?

Manage with triple assessment protocol including clinical assessment including history and physical examination. Image with ultrasound for those under 35 years plus mammogram for those over 35. Obtain a tissue sample with fine needle aspiration or core biopsy

EXAMINATION

Why is an ultrasound considered more useful than a mammogram in a younger patient?

The breast tissue is denser in the younger patient. Dense breasts have more fibrous and glandular tissue, which can appear white on a mammogram like a malignancy making a mammogram more difficult to interpret.

What are the complications of a mastectomy?

Immediate: Haemorrhage, nerve damage (intercostobrachial – T2), damage to long thoracic nerve of bell, thoracodorsal nerve damage, medial and lateral pectoral nerve damage.
Early: Infection, seroma, skin flap necrosis and asymmetry
Late: Lymphoedema, limitation of shoulder movement and psychological.

What are the levels associated with an axillary node clearance?

* Level I – Inferior to pectoralis minor (at lower edge)
* Level II – Posterior to pectoralis minor
* Level III – Medial / above to pectoralis minor
  (Note: The axillary25 artery is also divided according to its relation to pectoralis minor)

Outline the surface anatomy of the breast.

The breast overlies the 2nd to 6th ribs. Medially to lateral it runs form the lateral sternal edge to the mid axillary line. The breast tissue lies over the pectoralis major muscle with contributions from serratus anterior, external oblique and the superior aspect of the rectus sheath.

What is the arterial supply to the breast?

Internal thoracic, lateral thoracic and throracoacrominal arteries.

What are the boarders of the axillae?

The axilla is a pyramid shaped structure containing several important vessels and branches of the brachial plexus.
Medial wall – 1st to 4th ribs (with associated intercostal muscles and neurovascular bundles), serratus anterior
Lateral wall – Humerus (Bicipital groove)
Anteriorly – Pectoralis minor, pectoralis major, clavipectoral fascia
Posteriorly – Latissimus dorsi, scapula, subscapularis and teres major

What are the reconstruction options for a patient with breast cancer post mastectomy?

Reconstruction may be immediate or delayed. It may be prosthetic, autologous or a combination of the two.
Prosthetic – Insertion of an implant, either fixed volume or expandable
Expanders – Expand tissue over 3-6 months allowing for further reconstruction
Autologous –Movement of tissue from one area of the body to another with adequate blood supply to reconstruct the defect. Either in the form of a TRAM Flap (Trans Rectus Abdominus Myocutaneous Flap), DIEP Flap (Deep Inferior Epigastric Artery Perforator Flap) or a LD Flap (Latissimus Dorsi Flap).

What are the indications for mastectomy?

* Two or more tumours in the same breast

- Involvement of nipple-areolar complex
- DCIS (Ductal Cell Carcinoma in Situ)
- Genetic Predisposition (BRCA 1 & 2 positive)
- Patient preference
- Contraindication of radiotherapy or previous irradiation to breast tissue

What information is important from the histology report of a biopsy from potential breast cancer patients?

The specimen type (lymph node or breast tissue)
Macroscopic description
Microscopic description:
    The grade of the tumour (Grade 1-3)
    The size of the tumour
    The cell type
    Margin Clearance
    The invasion of the tumour cells (Lymphatic or vascular) and breech of the basement membrane.
    The presence of ER/ PR Receptors (Oestrogen Receptors/ Progesterone Receptors)
    The presence of HER2 Receptors (Human Epidermal Growth Factor Receptor 2)

What are Tamoxifen and Herceptin? What mechanism of action do they have?

Herceptin (Trastuzumab) is a monoclonal antibody, which targets human epidermal growth afctor HER2. Herceptin uses a mechanism called antibody dependent cellular cytoxicity to attract the hosts immune cells to the tumour site, where there is over expression of HER2 via.

Tamoxifen is a selective oestrogen receptor modulator (SERM) or antagonist. Tamoxifen acts as an anti-estrogen/inhibiting agent in the mammary tissue.

SUMMARY OF EXAMINATION

Wash Your Hands
Ensure that you are seen by the examiners to wash your hands using alcohol gel provided.

Introduce, Explain, Expose
Introduce yourself and check the identity of the patient. Expose adequately, ensuring chaperone present.

Inspect
Inspect with the patients hands over their head, and with hands pressed into waist.

Palpate
Palpate the four quadrants of the breast, nipple complex, tail of the pectoralis major muscle and the axillae. Check also for supraclavicular lymphadenopathy.
Palpate for liver and spine metastasis. Listen to the lung bases to examine for any lung metastasis.

Closing
Thank the patient. Inform them that they may now get dressed or ensure they are adequately covered.
Present your findings to the examiner.

TOP TIPS

➕ Always ensure a chaperone is asked for prior to starting the examination

➕ Ensure dignity of the patient throughout

➕ Don't forget to palpate for areas of breast metastasis at the end of the examination.

EXAMINATION

1.25 | Thyroid

Scenario

A 26-year-old male presents with a solitary lump on the anterior aspect of the neck. The lump is fixed to the underlying structures but moves with swallowing. There is a palpable lymph node in the anterior triangle of the neck. He reports having had previous radiotherapy to the right side of the neck.

Describe how you would begin

Expose and Inspect: Ask the patient to sit on a chair and inspect for any swellings sitting directly opposite the patient. Exposure the neck structures adequately, so the anterior and posterior triangles can be seen.

Ensure the patient is adequately positioned, sitting on a chair so you are able to examine the neck from the back.

Note any previous scars or, obvious eye signs or engorged neck veins from potential superior vena cava obstruction.

Note the clothes worn by the patient – are they appropriate for the ambient room temperature? Does the patient look anxious/sweaty/cold/tired?

EXAMINATION

Inspection Findings

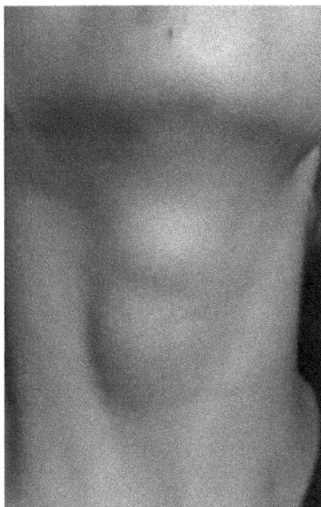

Describe what you see on inspection

On inspection there is a large nodule overlying the thyroid gland and extending onto the right hemi thyroid. The lump moves on swallowing. There is no evidence of SVC obstruction.

Having inspected what would you do next?

Thyroid Status Examination:
Hands
Inspect for a fine tremor (using a piece of paper over the hands), thyroid acropachy, palmar erythema, vitiligo, pulse (irregular? Tachycardia? Bradycardia?),

Eyes
Examine for lid retraction, exophalmos and proptosis by accessing from the front, above and sides of the patient. Proptosis is the forward displacment of an organ (not specifically the eye)
Exopthalmos is protrusion of they eyebll in their sockets from disease or injury.

Test for lid lag by asking the patient to follow your finger as it moves downwards quickly. Also test for diplopia by asking the patient to follow your finger as it makes the 'H' shape and test for visual acuity with a Snellen's chart.

Lower limb
Check for pre tibial myoedema and reflexes. Ask the patient to stand from a sitting position without using their arms to test for peripheral myopathy.

Thyroid Gland Examination:
Voice & swallowing:
Ask the patient to count from 1-10 accessing any hoarseness or airway impairment
Ask the patient to take a sip of water, retain it and observe the thyroid movement with swallowing
Ask the patient to protrude their tongue – checking for thyroglossal cyst

Palpation:
Palpate from behind the patient – warn them that you will do this
Palpate while the patient swallows and sticks out their tongue
Check if you can get beneath the gland itself
Examine each thyroid lobe in turn, examine for tenderness and temperature
Note the size, shape, nodularity and fixity of the lump
Palpate for tracheal deviation or displacement
Ask the patient to look left and right, tensing against your hand, accessing for the thyroids relationship to the sternocleidomastoid muscle.
Examine for regional lymph nodes

Percussion
Percuss the sternum to access for retrosternal goiter

Auscultate
Examine for thyroid bruits

> ### Findings
> On examination of the thyroid the lump is fixed and non-mobile, but smooth. The lump moves on swallowing.There is a palpable lymph node on the posterior boarder of the anterior triangle. Clinically the patient is euthyroid, with a heart rate of 85 bpm, and has a regular pulse. There is no retrosternal goitre evident on percussion, no bruits on auscultation and no evidence of superior vena cava obstruction.

What is your differential diagnosis?

A solitary nodule maybe due to:
- Thyroid cyst
- Adenoma/hyperplastic nodule
- Enlarged lobe (in Hashimoto's Thyroiditis)
- Primary malignancy – papillary, follicular, medullary or anaplastic carcinoma. Also lymphoma.

How would you manage this patient?

- Triple assessment of thyroid function tests, USS and FNA initially to guide further investigations and treatment.
- Patients with toxic nodules are usually managed under endocrinology – Tests include thyroid antibodies (thyroperoxidase (TPO), thyroglobulin (Tg) and TSH receptor) .
- If the patient was due to have surgery then preoperatively they need – clinicalhistory, examination and TFT, CXR, USS and radioisotope scanning. Laryngoscopy for vocal cord movements must be performed and documented before surgery
- The patient should be euthyroid prior to surgery. Thyrotoxicosis should be controlled with beta-blockers and carbimazole 2 weeks prior to surgery.

What are the structures traversed in a thyroidectomy from superficial to deep?

Skin, subcutaneous fat, superficial cervical fascia and platysma, deep investing layer of cervical fascia, strap muscles, pretracheal fascia, isthmus of thyroid.

What are the complications of a thyroidectomy?

Immediate
Recurrent laryngeal nerve damage
External laryngeal nerve damage – loss of high pitch
Early
Thyroid storm
Hypoparathyroidism and hypocalcaemia
Haematoma
Infection
Late
Scarring
Hypothyroidism

What are the sequelae of a) unilateral and b) bilateral recurrent laryngeal nerve palsy?

The recurrent laryngeal nerve is a branch of the vagus nerve. It supplies the intrinsic muscles of the larynx. If a unilateral paralysis occurs, the patient experiences a hoarse voice. If bilateral paralysis occurs, the patient experiences stridor and/or complete airway obstruction.

What is the blood supply to the thyroid gland?

The arterial supply is via the superior thyroid artery (from the external carotid artery) and the inferior thyroid artery (a branch of the thyrocervical trunk). In some patients, a third supply exists in the form of the thyroid ima artery, which is a branch directly from the aorta. The veins of the thyroid are the superior, middle and inferior thyroid veins. The latter drains into the brachiocephalic veins and the superior and middle thyroid veins drain into the internal jugular vein.

EXAMINATION

Why does the thyroid gland move with swallowing? Which ligament attaches the thyroid gland to the trachea?

The thyroid moves with swallowing because it is invested in the pre tracheal fascia and it is attached to the trachea by Berry's ligament. Berry's ligament attaches the thyroid to the trachea at the level of the 2nd to 4th tracheal rings.

SUMMARY OF EXAMINATION

Wash Your Hands
Ensure that you are seen by the examiners to wash your hands using alcohol gel provided.

Introduce, Explain, Expose and Inspect
Begin by introducing yourself, explain what you are going to do and check that this is ok with the patient and that he/she is not in any pain.
For thyroid examination, ensure adequate exposure of the neck

Inspect
Inspect for scars, neck swellings and any nodularity. Note the patients clothing.

Palpate
If there is a palpable lump assess the lump for fluctuance, size, shape, mobility/tethering. Access whether it is associated with the thyroid by asking the patient to swallow while palpating the lump. Access for any thyroglossal cysts by asking the patient to protrude their tongue.
Access the thyroid status by completion of the general examination, including skin changes, pulse, tremor, heart sounds and palpating for pre tibial myoedema.

Closing
Thank the patient. Inform them that they may now get dressed or ensure they are adequately covered.
Present your findings to the examiner.

1.26 | Peripheral Vascular

Scenario

Mr Ronald has been referred to the Vascular Surgery outpatient clinic by his GP with right calf pain on walking a distance of 50 metres. The patient is comfortable at rest. You have washed your hands and introduced yourself. Please perform a lower limb peripheral vascular examination.

Describe how you would begin

Wash hands and introduction: In particular, mention that you will need to palpate for pulses in the groin and that a chaperone will be present.

Expose and Inspect: The patient should be ideally exposed from abdomen to legs (including socks). Lie the patient supine at patient 45° and ensure that they are comfortable.

Inspect for skin changes, such as, pallor and mottling; trophic changes e.g. hair loss, thin skin and muscle atrophy, scars (suggestive of previous bypass procedures/vein harvest); areas of ulceration (look specifically between the toes and at the heel) and/or gangrene and amputations (ensure that you count all of the toes).

Inspection Findings

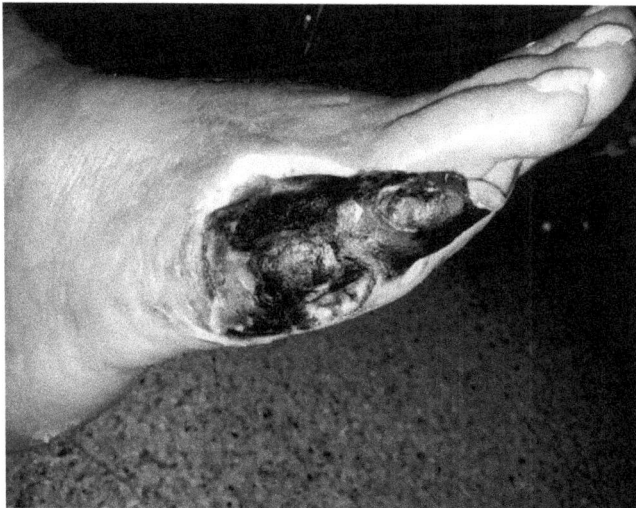

EXAMINATION

EXAMINATION

Describe what you see on inspection

On examination you identify a well demarcated area of dry necrosis affecting the right 5th toe.

Having inspected what would you do next?

Palpate

Feel for a temperature difference comparing both legs, using the back of your hands and starting distally to proximally.

Test capillary refill of the toes in each foot by pressing firmly for 5 seconds and measuring the time taken for refill to occur in seconds. This is normally <2 seconds.

In turn, palpate the pulses of the lower limb (femoral, popliteal, posterior tibial and dorsalis pedis). Compare both sides – assessing whether the pulses are equal on both sides, reduced or absent. A very easily palpable popliteal pulse should raise the suspicion of a popliteal aneurysm and you should specifically offer to assess for an abdominal aortic aneurysm. If bypass grafts are present palpate for pulsatility along its course (they may not be palpable if tunnelled deeply).

In acute limb ischaemia, the anterior, lateral and posterior muscle compartment should be assessed for tenderness (suggestive of compartment syndrome).

Auscultate

Listen for bruits in the iliac arteries (NB: that the aorta bifurcates at the level of L4, so, you should listen for a bruit in the line of the iliac artery inferior to the umbilicus) and femoral arteries (at the mid-inguinal point). The common femoral artery can also be auscultated in the groin and the superficial femoral artery at the adductor canal, which is one of the commonest sites of stenoses.

Special tests

Perform Buerger's test by slowly elevating the limb and observing Buerger's angle i.e. the angle at which the leg when elevated becomes pale. A Buerger's angle of less than 20 degrees indicates severe ischaemia. The foot is then placed over the edge of the bed and the foot assessed for the appearance of reactive hyperaemia. If reactive hyperaemia is present, this is a positive Buerger's test.

> ### ᘒᘒᑎ Findings
>
> The right lower limb is cooler to the midfoot compared to the left. Femoral pulses can be palpated bilaterally, however, no popliteal pulse or foot pulses can be are palpated in the right lower limb. They are palpable on the left. Buerger's test is positive on the right, with a Buerger's angle of 20 degrees. This would be keeping with severe right limb ischaemia.

What is your differential diagnosis?

The differential diagnosis for intermittent claudication includes:
- Arterial causes, which may be due to:
• Thrombosis i.e. atherosclerosis
• Embolic - atrial fibrillation, AAA, coagulopathy
- Neurological causes e.g. spinal stenosis, lumbar nerve root irritation
- Musculoskeletal causes e.g. osteoarthritis of the hip/knee

Given the examination findings, the most likely diagnosis is severe limb ischaemia of the right lower limb due to significant peripheral vascular disease.

How would you manage this patient?

Management should include taking a full history, a complete examination and the appropriate investigations. This will determine the definitive management plan.

Options for treatment include:
• Conservative management with best medical management (BMT) (e.g. smoking cessation, encouraging exercise, statin and anti-platelet therapy, optimisation of diabetes, blood pressure etc.,).
• Surgical interventional: this may be by percutaneous intervention (angioplasty) or open surgical (bypass grafting).

Key points when considering surgical intervention in chronic limb ischaemia, include:
• The extent to which the patients' symptoms limit their activities of daily living and whether optimal conservative management has been achieved.
• The presence of rest pain or tissue loss (i.e. severe limb ischaemia).
• Co-morbidities that may preclude intervention.

How would you determine the level of the vascular lesion?

The clinical examination can help identify the level of the lesion, for example, an absent femoral pulse indicates disease proximal to the common femoral artery (i.e. within iliac arteries).

How would you determine the aetiology of the claudication?

Warm lower limbs and palpable pulses would suggest a neurological cause for the claudication. A straight leg raise may also be positive.

What is atherosclerosis?

Atherosclerosis is the remodelling of the arterial wall secondary to plaque formation.

There are four main stages: initial damage to the vascular endothelium and deposition of intracellular lipids (fatty streak), accumulation of inflammatory cells and ingestion of fat molecules (foam cells), proliferation of smooth muscle cells secondary to persistent inflammation, followed by the formation of a fibrous cap between the fatty deposits and vascular intima (mature plaque).

What classification system is used to determine severity of peripheral vascular disease?

The Fontaine classification system is used to determine the severity of peripheral vascular disease.

Stage I: Asymptomatic
Stage II: Intermittent claudication; IIa) can walk >200m, IIb) <200m
Stage III: Rest pain
Stage IV: Tissue loss (ulceration or gangrene)

EXAMINATION

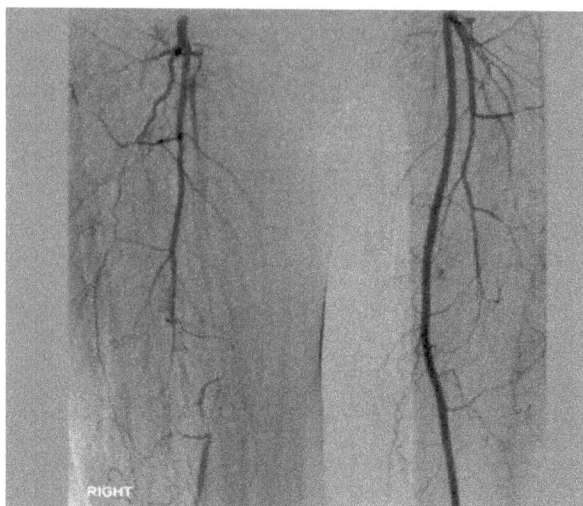

What does the angiogram demonstrate?

This catheter angiogram of the lower limb vascular tree demonstrates an occluded right superficial femoral artery from its origin, which reconstitutes distally via collaterals. This is commonly due to the narrowing of the artery as it passes through the adductor hiatus.

SUMMARY OF EXAMINATION

Wash Your Hands
Ensure that you are seen by the examiners to wash your hands using the alcohol gel provided.

Introduce, Explain, Expose and Inspect
Begin by introducing yourself, explain what you are going to do and check that this is ok with the patient and that he/she is not in any pain (particularly in the hip as you will be performing Buerger's test). The patient should ideally be wearing only underwear.

Patient Position
Sitting on couch at 45°.

Inspect
For skin changes, trophic changes, tissue loss, previous amputation and vascular surgical scars.

Palpate
Assess temperature of both limbs and capillary refill. Palpate all lower limb pulses in turn, comparing both sides.

Auscultate
For bruits in the iliac and femoral arteries.

Special tests
Perform Buerger's test by slowly elevating the limb and observing Buerger's angle i.e. the angle at which the leg when elevated becomes pale. A Buerger's angle of less than 20

EXAMINATION

degrees indicates severe ischaemia. The foot is then placed over the edge of the bed and the foot assessed for the appearance of reactive hyperaemia. If reactive hyperaemia is present, this is a positive Buerger's test.

Closing
Thank the patient. Inform them that they may now get dressed or ensure they are adequately covered.
Present your findings to the examiner.

Complete examination by performing an abdominal examination to exclude the presence of an AAA, a neurological lower limb assessment, full cardiovascular system examination, ABPI's and lower limb arterial doppler ultrasound scan.

TOP TIPS

➕ Ensure to count toes on each foot, it is very easy to miss a well-healed toe amputation site.

➕ Practice palpating normal pulses before the exam – it can be easy to mistake your own pulse for that of the patient in a stressful exam setting.

➕ Palpating the abdomen is essential to exclude an AAA. This can contribute to lower limb pathology (*e.g. due to an embolic phenomenon).*

EXAMINATION

1.27 | Prostate

Scenario

Mr Smith presents to the surgical outpatient clinic with difficulty passing urine for the past few months. You would like to perform a PR examination to examine the prostate. The patient is comfortable. You have washed your hands, introduced yourself and explained what you are going to do. Please perform a digital rectal examination (DRE).

Describe how you would begin

Wash hands and introduction: Discuss with the patient the nature of the exam, reasons for needing to perform an invasive examination and that a chaperone will be present. Gain verbal consent to the examination.

Expose and Inspect: Position the patient in the left lateral position with knees as far up to the abdomen as possible. Inspect the perianal region for lesions e.g. sentinel skin tags.

Findings

On inspection there is a benign skin tag at 3 o'clock in the perianal region.

Having inspected what would you do next?

Palpate

First test perianal sensation with a gloved finger. Warn the patient prior to performing the internal aspect of the digital rectal examination. Ensure that you use a sufficient amount of KY jelly.

Palpate methodically all of the zones of the prostate (central and peripheral). Assess for size, consistency and surface. When palpating the prostate gland ask the patient if they feel any pain. Determine the absence of any rectal lesions and mucosal abnormalities. On removal of your finger, assess for the presence of blood (fresh or maleana).

Findings

The prostate is diffusely enlarged, non-tender and has a smooth surface. No rectal lesions were identified.

What is your differential diagnosis?

Possible differential diagnoses include:
• Benign prostatic hyperplasia (BPH)
• Prostate cancer
• Prostatitis
The most likely aetiology in this case is BPH due to the findings of a smooth, non-tender prostate.

How would you manage this patient?

Management involves taking a full history and examining the patient. Investigations include PSA and if the PSA is elevated, a transrectal ultrasound (TRUS) and biopsy is indicated to exclude malignancy. If a malignancy is confirmed, a CT thorax/abdomen/pelvis is required for cancer staging, as well as an isotope bone scan to exclude bone metastases.

Management of BPH includes medical therapy (e.g. α-Blockers) or surgical treatment, which is indicated if medical therapy has failed or if the patient is experiencing severe symptoms.

How can you differentiate between the above possible diagnoses?

In prostatitis, the prostate is smoothly enlarged and tender; whilst in BPH, the prostate is non-tender and a median groove can be palpated. In prostatic cancer the prostate gland feels asymmetrical, firm or nodular.

Describe the anatomical position of the prostate and its relationship to surrounding structures

The prostate lies on the urogenital diaphragm with the urethra and ejaculatory ducts running through its tissue. The bladder is superior, pubis bone anterior, with the rectum and seminal vesicles lying posteriorly to the prostate

What is the Gleason grading system?

The Gleason grade represents the architectural changes seen on prostatic biopsies under microscopy in prostatic cancer. The two most common Gleason grades (1-5) seen are added together to give a total score (2-10), with a higher score representing a more poorly differentiated tumour. It can be used to predict prognosis together with other factors such as PSA.

Why does prostatic cancer metastasise to the vertebrae?

The Batson venous plexus are valveless veins that connect the venous drainage of the prostate to the internal vertebral venous plexus. Due to the absence of valves, it can provide a route for the metastaic spread of prostatic cancer cells to the vertebral bodies.

In which patient group would you offer radical prostatectomy?

This is controversial and is dependant on patient wishes, disease state and life expectancy. Ideal candidates have few co-morbidities, local disease confined to the prostate (T1-2) and impotence is not important to the patient (this is a common complication).

What is TURP syndrome and how is it managed?

TURP syndrome is a collection of symptoms which occur as a result of absorption of the irrigation fluid used during a TURP procedure via the prostatic vasculature. This can lead to hyponatraemia and encephalopathy (secondary to the metabolism of glycine into ammonia). Risk factors for TURP syndrome include length of the operation, general anaesthetic (cannot identify the early signs of confusion), large prostates and glycine-containing irrigation fluid. Management is mainly supportive, including fluid restriction and diuretic therapy.

EXAMINATION

SUMMARY OF EXAMINATION

Wash Your Hands
Ensure that you are seen by the examiners to wash your hands using the alcohol gel provided.

Introduce, Explain, Expose and Inspect
Begin by introducing yourself, explain what you are going to do to the patient and explain that a chaperone will be present throughout the examination.

Patient Position
Position the patient in the left lateral position with hips and knees as fully flexed as possible. Ensure patient the is covered until the digital rectal examination is performed.

Inspect
For perianal lesions e.g. skin tags, fissures, sinuses.

Palpate
Assess the size of the prostate gland, palpating each lobe individually, together with its surface and consistency. Determine whether there is any tenderness on palpation.

Closing
Assist the patient to a seated position and thank the patient. Inform them that they may now get dressed and you will discuss the examination findings with them after this. Present your findings to the examiner.

Complete the examination by performing an abdominal examination and palpating for spinal tenderness.

TOP TIPS

➕ Always make sure you say that a chaperone will be present throughout the examination.

➕ Taking time to place the patient in the correct position makes it less awkward for the patient during the PR examination and provides adequate exposure in order to assess the prostate gland fully.

➕ Ensure you appreciate the different lobes of the prostate and their likely pathology.

1.28 | Testicular

Scenario

Mr Bracken presents to the acute surgical admissions unit with a tender, swollen testicle. The patient is comfortable at rest. You have washed your hands, introduced yourself and explained what you are going to do. Please perform a testicular examination.

Describe how you would begin

Wash hands and introduction: Particularly mention that you will need to examine both the groin and testicles, but that a chaperone will be present throughout. Gain verbal consent to the examination.

Expose and Inspect: The patient should remove their trousers and underwear, and lie supine. Keep the patient covered until you are ready to start the examination.

Inspect for any skin changes, testicular or groin swellings, an absent testes (e.g. maldescended or absent), previous scars (e.g. from an orchidectomy or scrotal incision) and whether a cough impulse is present.

👓 Findings

On examination you identify a grossly swollen right testicle. There is no evidence of previous surgery in the region and no cough impulse.

Having inspected what would you do next?

Palpate
Feel for an increase in temperature of the testicles. Assess for any swelling within the testicle describing their site (i.e. skin, epididymis, spermatic cord, testes), size, surface, consistency and whether you can get above the swelling. Also discern whether the testicle is tender and whether there is an associated cough impulse/if the swelling is reducible.

Special tests
Transilluminate the swelling with a pen torch.
Palpate for lymphadenopathy in the inguinal region.

👓 Findings

The swelling measures 4 x 3 cm, has a smooth surface and is indistinct from the testes. It is tender on palpation. There is no cough impulse and it does not transilluminate. There are enlarged, smooth lymph nodes in the right inguinal region.

What is your differential diagnosis?

Use a surgical sieve and think of the potential structures that could be involved in this region:
• Skin – scrotal oedema, sebaceous cyst

EXAMINATION

- Testes – hydrocoele, haematocoele, testicular torsion
- Epididymis – epididymal cyst, acute/chronic epidiymitis
- Venous – varicocoele
- Inflammatory/infective – acute orchitis
- Hernia – inguino-scrotal
- Lymphoma

Given the examination findings, the most likely diagnosis is epididymo-orchitis.

How would you manage this patient?

Management should involve taking a full history and performing an abdominal examination. Investigations include urine cultures, together with urethral swabs (testing for chlamydia and gonorrhoea) and are required prior to starting treatment. Simple measures such as the elevation of the scrotum with a scrotal support and cold packs will produce symptomatic relief. Appropriate simple analgesia and antibiotics should be prescribed, as per local protocol.

How does your examination help to differentiate between the differential diagnoses above?

Clinically if you cannot get above the swelling the most likely diagnosis is an inguino-scrotal hernia. Therefore, you should then ask the patient to reduce the hernia back into the inguinal canal and determine the position of the abdominal wall defect.

A swelling which trans-illuminates is most likely to be a hydrocoele, while a tender swelling implies the possibility of an inflammatory/infective aetiology.

Why does the scrotal skin have a wrinkled appearance?

This is due to the dartos fascia being adherent to the scrotal skin, with the fascia's smooth muscle being responsible for the wrinkled appearance. The dartos fascia is continuous with the Scarpa's fascia of the abdomen.

Describe the lymphatic drainage of the testicle

- The testes drains into the para-aortic nodes.
- The scrotum drains to the superficial inguinal nodes.

What are the contents of the spermatic cord?

Remember the rule of threes:

- Three arteries: Artery to vas, cremasteric and testicular arteries
- Three veins: Pampiniform plexus, cremasteric and testicular veins
- Three fascial coverings: External spermatic (from external oblique), cremasteric (internal oblique and transversus abdominus) and internal spermatic (transversalis fascia) fascia
- Three nerves: Sympathetic nerves, genital branch of genitofemoral nerve and ilioinguinal nerve
- Three other structures: Vas, processus vaginalis and lymphatics

What blood tests are required if an ultrasound scan demonstrates a testicular tumour?

Most testicular tumours arise from the germ cells of the testes and generally are either seminomas or non-seminomatous germ cell tumours - NSGCT), such as teratomas. Blood tumour markers aid in diagnosis, response to treatment and surveillance post-treatment.

These include:
• β-HCG – raised in NSGCT and some seminomas
• Alpha-fetoprotein (α-FP) – may be raised in NSGCT. Not raised in seminomas.
• LDH – useful to assess tumour load

How do you perform an orchidectomy for testicular cancer?

• After a full history, thorough examination and relevant investigations, formal written consent is obtained.
• The correct testicle for surgery is marked.
• Appropriate tumour markers are sent pre-operatively.
• The procedure is performed under general anaesthesia. The patient is placed in a supine position and prepped and draped in the standard fashion.
• An incision is performed 2cm above the inguinal ligament (using surface markings) and extended down through subcutaneous tissue and fascia towards the inguinal canal.
• The inguinal canal is entered by incising the external oblique aponeurotic fibres and extending the incision to the superficial ring.
• The ilioinguinal nerve is identified and preserved.
• The spermatic cord is dissected to the deep inguinal ring and clamped.
• The testicle is delivered from the scrotum, while ligating the scrotal attachments. The testicle is then inspected.
• Each component of the cord at the deep ring is dissect out and ligated.
• The incision is closed in layers.

SUMMARY OF EXAMINATION

EXAMINATION

Wash Your Hands
Ensure that you are seen by the examiners to wash your hands using the alcohol gel provided.

Introduce, Explain, Expose and Inspect
Begin by introducing yourself, explain what you are going to do and that a chaperone will be present throughout the examination.

Patient Position
Supine.

Inspect
For skin changes, scars, swellings and previous orchidectomy. Assess for the presence of a cough impulse.

Palpate
Assess temperature of both testicles and whether a swelling is present. Describe the swelling in relation to testicular structures if possible and whether you can get above the swelling. Determine the presence of a cough impulse and whether the swelling is reducible.

Special tests
Transilluminate the swelling and palpate the inguinal region for the presence of lymphadenopathy.

Closing
Thank the patient. Inform them that they may now get dressed or ensure they are

adequately covered.
Present your findings to the examiner.

TOP TIPS

➕ Take your time and attempt to determine which structures are distinct from the swelling.

➕ Always assess for the presence of a cough impulse and perform a groin examination if this is present.

➕ In young patients with a short history of testicular swelling always consider a diagnosis of testicular torsion.

1.29 | Ulcer

Scenario

Mrs Hughes has been referred to the surgical outpatient clinic with an ulcer on her left leg. She is comfortable at rest. You have washed your hands, introduced yourself and explained what you are going to do. Please perform an examination of her lower leg ulcer.

Describe how you would begin

Wash hands and introduction: Mention that a chaperone will be present throughout the examination and ask the patient if they have any pain in their hips.

Expose and inspect: Patient to remove clothing (including socks) down to underwear. Place patient lying on couch at 45 degrees.

Observe for any skin changes suggestive of arterial or venous disease, tissue loss, varicose veins, scars (suggestive of previous bypass procedures/vein harvest or trauma) and amputations (ensure you count toes). Ensure you lift the patient's leg to inspect the posterior aspect of both lower limbs.

Identify the presence of an ulcer and describe the ulcer according to its:

- **Site**
- **Size**
- **Shape** – e.g. irregular, round
- **Edge** – e.g. everted, punched out
- **Base** – e.g. sloughy, necrotic, with healthy granulation tissue. Determine if any structures can be seen at the base (e.g. muscle, tendon, bones) together with the presence of any discharge (serous, haemoserous, purulent).
- **Depth** – e.g. shallow
- **Surrounding Tissue**

Findings

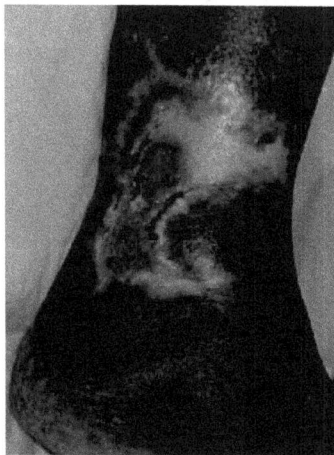

EXAMINATION

Describe what you see on inspection

On inspection, there is an irregular 5cm x 8cm ulcer overlying the medial aspect of the left leg. It has shallow sloping edges and a granulating base. There are associated venous skin changes of lipodermatosclerosis and the ulcer is painful.

Having inspected what would you do next?

Palpate

Assess for sensation in the skin surrounding the ulcer - if there is no sensation present proceed to perform a lower limb neurological examination. In addition, palpate for peripheral pulses. In the case above, the most likely aetiology of the ulcer is venous. Therefore offer to examine specifically for varicose veins.

Special tests

Assess for lymphadenopathy in the inguinal region bilaterally and offer to perform ABPIs. The latter is important when treating venous ulcers.

> ### ᓚ Findings
>
> There is normal sensation in the skin surrounding the ulcer and foot pulses are present bilaterally.

What is your differential diagnosis?

Use a surgical sieve and think of the potential structures that could be involved in this region:
• Vascular - arterial, venous or mixed
• Neuropathic/neuroischaemic - diabetic ulcer
• Malignant – Marjolin's ulcer, SCC, BCC
• Inflammatory/infective – dermatomyositis, pyoderma gangrenosum
• Trauma
Given the examination findings, the most likely diagnosis is venous ulceration.

How would you manage this patient?

An arterial component to the ulcer should be excluded and if the ulcer has a mixed arterial-venous component, the arterial disease should be corrected. Investigations (venous and arterial duplex imaging) will help in determining the aetiology of the ulcer if it is not immediately apparent. Further management includes:

Non-Surgical
• Rest and elevate the leg to reduce leg swelling
• Four layer compression bandaging (Note ABPIs should be greater than 0.9) for this degree of compression dressing).
• Once healed, the patient should wear Class II compression hosiery.
• Antibiotics may be indicated if the ulcer is clearly infected.

Surgical
• Exclude malignancy - either a punch or excisional biopsy can be used to determine sinister pathology
• Skin grafting if clean
• Treat primary varicose vein

How do the examination findings differentiate between the potential aetiology of the ulcer?

Arterial ulcers have a 'punched-out' appearance, are painful, affect distal extremities and are associated with absent peripheral pulses. They often have a deep base that often lacks granulation tissue and may be necrotic (see picture below).

Venous ulcers typically have sloping and shallow edges, affect the gaiter area of the leg and are associated with signs of venous hypertension. They are usually painful and can be large and are irregular.

Neuropathic ulcers are seen over pressure areas and have even wound margins and there is often callous formation around the ulcer. They are typically painless and peripheral pulses are present, unless there is co-existing peripheral vascular disease (i.e. the ulcer is neuro-ischaemic) (see picture below).

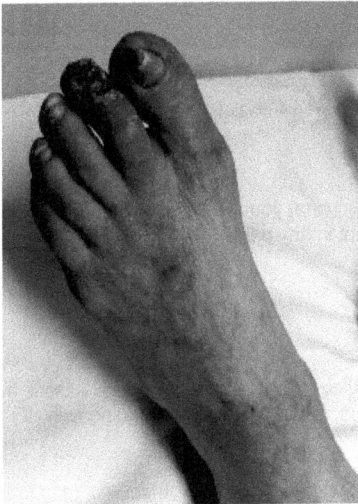

Arterial ulcer affecting distal extremities

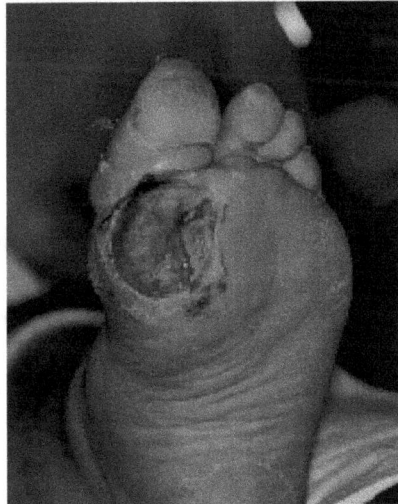

Neuropathic ulcer affecting ball of foot

EXAMINATION

What is the definition of an ulcer?

A break in the continuity of an epithelial surface (either skin or a mucous membrane).

What is a Marjolin's ulcer?

A Marjolin's ulcer is an aggressive ulcerating squamous cell carcinoma that commonly appears at the site of previous traumatised or chronically inflamed skin.

How would you manage a venous ulcer?

Management of the causal factor is paramount to allow for the healing of the ulcer and prevention of further lesions developing. Treatment of any infection present and compression bandaging form the cornerstone of treatment. Definitive treatment of varicose veins should also be considered, using either endovenous ablation techniques, foam sclerotherapy and less commonly, high-tie of the sapheno-femoral junction and stripping of the long saphenous vein or sapheno-popliteal junction ligation.

How would you manage an arterial ulcer?

Management can be either medical or surgical.
Medical
- Analgesia
- Optimisation of cardiovascular risk factors
- Antibiotics, if infection is present
- Wound care

Surgical
- Debridement – this may surgical or non-surgical e.g. larvae
- Improve blood supply e.g. angioplasty, bypass grafting
- Amputation – may be indicated if the limb is deemed unsalvageable.

From which cell does a basal cell carcinoma originate?

This originates from the basal cells of the epidermis.

SUMMARY OF EXAMINATION

Wash Your Hands
Ensure that you are seen by the examiners to wash your hands using the alcohol gel provided.

Introduce, Explain, Expose and Inspect
Begin by introducing yourself to the patient. Explain what you are going to do and check that this is ok with the patient and that he/she is not in any pain.

Patient Position
Sitting on a couch at 45 degrees.

Inspect
For skin changes, varicose veins, tissue loss, previous amputations and scars. Assess the ulcer for the following: site, size, shape, edge, base, depth and the surrounding skin.

Palpate
Assess the temperature of each limb and around the ulcer (indicating infection). In addition, assess for loss of sensation around the ulcer.

Special tests
Assess for lymphadenopathy in the inguinal region and palpate peripheral pulses.

Closing
Thank the patient. Inform them that they may now get dressed or ensure they are adequately covered.
Present your findings to the examiner.

Complete your examination by performing a neurovascular examination of the lower limbs and a varicose vein examination, if appropriate. Request a lower limb venous and arterial Doppler ultrasound scan, if relevant.

1.30 | Varicose Veins

Scenario

Mrs Jones presents to the surgical outpatient clinic with varicose veins, which have been symptomatic for over a year. The patient is comfortable at rest. You have washed your hands, introduced yourself to the patient and explained what you are going to do. Please examine this patient's varicose veins.

Describe how you would begin

Wash hands and introduction: Particularly mention that you will need to palpate for a groin swelling and that a chaperone will be present.

Expose and Inspect: All the patients clothing below the waist down should be removed (not including underwear but including socks). The patient should be standing.

Observe for any skin changes (venous eczema, pigmentation, lipodermatosclerosis or ulceration), varicose veins (including their distribution in lower limb), swellings (in the groins), oedema and scars (suggestive of vein harvest, previous venous surgery or healed ulcers).

Inspection Findings

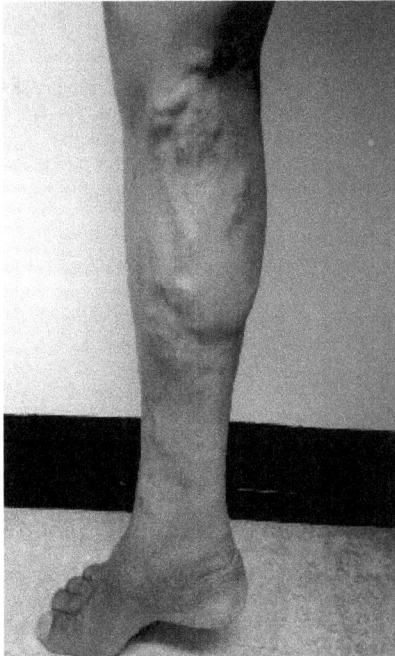

EXAMINATION

Describe what you see on inspection

On inspection you find varicose veins in both legs, predominantly on the medial aspect. There is evidence of venous eczema.

Having inspected what would you do next?

Palpate

Palpate the varicosities along their entire course, assessing for tenderness, temperature and lumpiness suggestive of thrombophlebitis. Palpate each sapheno-femoral junction in turn (4 cm inferiorly and lateral to the pubic tubercle) to determine the presence of a saphena varix. This is a soft swelling which has a blue discolouration and will transmit a cough impulse (see picture below).

Auscultate

Listen for bruits at the saphenofemoral junction to determine the presence of an arteriovenous fistula (this may be iatrogenic e.g. secondary to femoral arterial puncture).

Special tests

Perform the following tests:

• Tap test: Place two fingers over a varicose vein and tap the varicosity more proximally using two fingers of the other hand. If a transmitted impulse is felt in the distal two fingers, this indicates valvular incompetence.

• Trendelenberg test: With the patient supine, elevate one leg. Milk the veins empty proximally using your other hand and manually compress the sapheno-femoral junction. Maintaining pressure at the sapheno-femoral junction, ask the patient to stand. If the patient's varicose veins do not reappear on standing, this suggests that the sapheno-femoral junction is incompetent. Repeat this test for the other leg.

•Tourniquet test: With the patient supine, elevate one leg. Milk the veins empty proximally using your other hand and place a tourniquet as high as possible around the thigh. Then ask the patient to stand. If the varicose veins do not reappear, the level of incompetence is at or above the level of the tourniquet. If the varicose veins do reappear, repeat the test again with the tourniquet at the level of the mid-thigh and so-forth, until the varicose veins are controlled.

•Perthe's test: With the patient supine, elevate one leg. Milk the veins empty proximally using your other hand and place a tourniquet at the level of the sapheno-femoral junction to occlude the superficial venous pathway. Ask the patient to repeatedly stand up and down on their tiptoes for at least one minute. If the patient experiences pain this suggests deep venous incompetence.

•Hand-held Doppler: Place the Doppler probe over the sapheno-femoral junction and squeeze the calf muscle of the same limb. A 'whoosh' sound with an abrupt cut-off corresponds to a competent junction. If the 'whoosh' is followed by a further 'whoosh' then junction is incompetent. Perform this test at both the sapheno-femoral and sapheno–popliteal junctions in each limb.

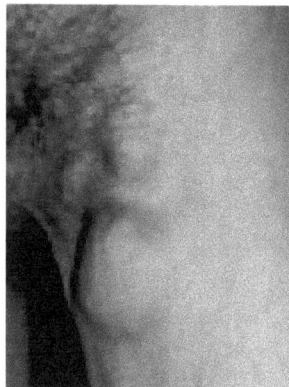

> ### 〰️ Findings
>
> There are varicose veins in the distribution of the long saphenous bilaterally. The tap test was positive. The tourniquet test demonstrated that the level of incompetence was at the sapheno-femoral junctions. A sapheno-varix was seen on the left. In summary, this patient has varicose veins secondary to bilateral sapheno-femoral junction incompetence.

What are varicose veins?

Varicose veins can be defined as tortuous, dilated, elongated veins of the superficial venous system.

What symptoms do patients with varicose veins report?

* Cosmesis
* Leg aching
* Leg swelling and/or heaviness
* Cramping
* Itchiness
* Bleeding
* Venous skin changes e.g. eczema, lipodermatosclerosis
* Venous ulceration

How would you manage this patient?

This patient has symptomatic varicose veins and therefore meets NICE Guidelines (2013) for treatment. Formal venous Doppler ultrasound is required to confirm the diagnosis of varicose veins and the extent of truncal reflux, and to plan treatment. In addition, I would give advice regarding weight loss, light to moderate exercise, leg elevation and avoidance of factors that make the patient's symptoms worse.

If varicose veins and truncal reflux is confirmed on venous duplex imaging:

* I would offer endothermal ablation.
* If endothermal ablation is unsuitable, I would offer ultrasound-guided foam sclerotherapy.
* If ultrasound-guided foam sclerotherapy is unsuitable, I would offer surgery.

I would not offer compression hosiery to treat varicose veins unless interventional treatment was unsuitable.

What are the complications of endovenous ablation treatment of varicose veins?

* Bleeding/bruising
* Thromboembolic events i.e. Deep vein thrombosis and pulmonary embolism
* Nerve damage e.g. thermal injury to the saphenous or sural nerve
* Skin burns – this is usually due to inadequate tumescent anaesthesia and can result in skin discolouration or ulceration

• Recurrence

SUMMARY OF EXAMINATION

Wash Your Hands

Ensure that you are seen by the examiners to wash your hands using the alcohol gel provided.

Introduce, Explain, Expose and Inspect

Begin by introducing yourself, explain what you are going to do and check that this is ok with the patient and that he/she is not in any pain (particularly in the hips as you will be performing the tournique/Trendelenberg's test). The patient should ideally be wearing only underwear in their lower half.

Patient Position

The patient should be standing.

Inspect

For skin changes, varicosities, a saphenovarix in the groin, ulcers and scars.

Palpate

Palpate the varicosities and assess for the presence of a sapheno-varix.

Special tests

Tap-test, tourniquet test, Trendelenberg test, Perthe's test and hand-held Doppler (see above).

Closing

Thank the patient. Inform them that they may now get dressed or ensure they are adequately covered.

Present your findings to the examiner.

Complete your examination by performing a peripheral vascular examination of the lower limbs, an abdominal examination to exclude the presence of an intra-abdominal mass and a venous Doppler ultrasound scan.

TOP TIPS

➕ Practice makes perfect – the special tests can be tricky to perform ad hoc as they require specific patient positioning and explanation

➕ The Doppler test is simple but knowledge of the sapheno-femoral junction surface anatomy is key.

➕ Ensure you know what you should hear in a normal and abnormal Doppler test.

2 SURGICAL SKILLS

2.1 Arterial Blood Gas 156
2.2 ATLS Survey 160
2.3 Blood Taking 163
2.4 Cannulation 165
2.5 Central Line 168
2.6 Chest Drain 171
2.7 Wound Debridement 175
2.8 Discharge/Transfer Summary 178
2.9 Fine Needle Aspiration 180
2.10 Knee Joint Aspiration 183
2.11 Knot Tying 187
2.12 Local Anaesthetic 190
2.13 Lumbar Puncture 193
2.14 Male Urethral Catheterisation 197
2.15 Needle Thoracostomy 201
2.16 Organising a List A 206
2.17 Organising a List B 212
2.18 Removal of a Naevus 218
2.19 Scrubbing Up 223
2.20 Suturing 226

SURGICAL SKILLS

SURGICAL SKILLS

2.1 | Arterial Blood Gas

Scenario

You are the CT2 on the general surgery ward. A 65 male patient has been admitted with acute pancreatitis yesterday. You receive a call from the FY1 who has taken an arterial blood gas as part of the work up, as the patient is tachycardic, tachypnoeic, desaturating and febrile.

The results are as follows:

pH 7.31

paO2 on 2L O²: 8.2 kpA

paCO²: 4.1 kpA

HCO³: 11 mmol per L

BE: +4.2

Anion gap: 18

Lactate: 6

What does the blood gas show?
Uncompensated metabolic acidosis with elevated serum lactate

What is the 'base excess'?

Base excess is the amount of acid or alkali (base) required to restore 1 litre of blood to a normal pH at a PaCO2 of 5.4kPa at 37 degrees celcius

Normal range is −2 to +2mmol per litre.

Define the term pH

The pH is the $-\log 10$ [H+]

What are the main buffers in the plasma, interstitial and intercellular compartments

• Plasma
   o Bicarbonate system
   o Plasma proteins
   o Haemoglobin
   o Phosphate system
• Intracellular
   o Cytoplasmic proteins
• Interstitial
   o Bicarbonate system

What is the Henderson-Hasselbach equation
This equation is used to describe the equilibrium of the bicarbonate buffer system:

$$CO_2 + H_2O = H_2CO_3 = HCO_3^- + H^+$$

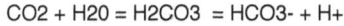

How do you manage a patient with this acid-base disturbance (metabolic lactic acidosis)

Management of underlying cause:
- E.g. IV fluid for shock, emergency dialysis for renal failure, inotropic support for cardiac output to counteract poor tissue perfusion
- IV bicarbonate is controversial
-

Which organs are involved in regulating acid-base balance

i. Kidneys – by regulating bicarbonate, long-term control
ii. Lungs – hyperventilation can blow off CO_2 and increases pH. Hypoventilation conserves CO_2 and decreases pH
iii. Blood – by plasma proteins and haemoglobin

SUMMARY

Use a relevant system to interpret an ABG. Look at the pH and decide if there is an alkalosis or an acidosis. Be aware that if the pH is normal, this may indicate compensation. Next look at the $PaCO_2$ which may be high indicating a respiratory acidosis or compensation of a metabolic alkalosis. If the $PaCO_2$ is low, this may indicate a respiratory acidosis or metabolic compensation. Next, look at the HCO_3^- and if it is high, this indicates metabolic alkalosis or compensation of a respiratory acidosis. If it is low, this suggests a metabolic acidosis or respiratory alkalosis compensation.

Equipment Required
- ABG Pack:
- A blue (23 G) needle
- 2ml syringe with heparin
- a cap for the syringe
- a plastic bung
- Alcohol wipe
- Gauze
- Gloves
- Sharps bin

Introuduce, Gain Consent and Assess Perfusion
Locate the radial artery with your index and middle fingers. Perform an Allen's test where you compress both the radial and ulnar arteries at the same time. The hand should become white, then release the ulnar artery and the colour should return to the hand. This ensures that there will still be a blood supply to the hand should the ABG cause a blockage in the radial artery.

Prepare ABG Kit
Put on your gloves and attach the needle to the heparinised syringe.

Take Arterial Blood
Let the patient know you are about to proceed and to expect a sharp scratch.
Insert the needle at 30 degrees to the skin at the point of maximum pulsation of the radial artery. Advance the needle until arterial blood flushes into the syringe. The arterial pressure will cause the blood to fill the syringe.

Remove the needle/syringe placing the needle into the bung. Press firmly over the

SURGICAL SKILLS

puncture site with the gauze to halt the bleeding. Remain pressed for up to 5 minutes to ensure haemostasis.

Disposal and Finishing
Remove the needle and discard safely in the sharps bin. Cap the syringe, push out any air within it, and send immediately for analysis ensuring that the sample is packed in ice. Remove your gloves and dispose them in the clinical waste bin. Wash your hands and thank the patient.

Analysis and Interpretation
The syringe should be carefully trasnported to an ABG machine and the results interpreted.

Metabolic Acidosis	Respiratory Acidosis
pH: Low	pH: Low
pCO2: =	pCO2: High
Bicarbonate: Low	Bicarbonate: =
Metabolic Alkalosis	**Respiratory Alkalosis**
pH: High	pH: High
pCO2: =	pCO2: Low
Bicarbonate: High	Bicarbonate: =

TOP TIPS

➕ Don't forget to look at all of the ABG results and not just the information relevant to acid base – you may miss an Hb of 4 in a bleeding patient, or a glucose of 2 in an unresponsive, hypoglycaemic patient!

2.2 | ATLS Assessment

Scenario

You are the orthopaedic SHO on call at the weekend. You receive a trauma call to A&E Resus where an unresponsive 30-year-old man has been admitted following a head on car crash into a parked vehicle. He arrives at hospital via basic life support with cervical collar in situ and strapped to a backboard.

How would you perform a primary survey on this patient?

Airway with cervical spine protection
• Ascertain airway patency and assess for airway obstruction
• Assume C spine with blunt multisystem trauma, altered consciousness, blunt injury above clavicle

Breathing
• Expose
• Inspect
• Auscultate
• Palpate
• Percuss
• Use adjunctd e.g. pulse oximetry and arterial blood gas (ABG)

Circulation with haemorrhage control
• Blood volume and cardiac output
• Identify source of external, extrasanguinating haemorrhage
• Identify internal bleeding e.g. chest, abdomen, retroperitoneum, pelvis and long bones identified by physical examination and imaging e.g. CXR, pelvic x-ray or focused assessment sonography (FAST).
• Skin colour
• Pulse
• Level of consciousness
• Use adjuncts such as blood pressure, ECG, gastric or urinary catheters

Disability (neurologic evaluation)
• GCS
• Pupillary size and reaction
• Level of consciousness
• Lateralising signs
• Spinal cord injury level

Environmental including hypothermia
• Fully expose the patient, usually by cutting off garments
• Ensure warm environment
• Warm IVF
• Use adjuncts e.g. Chest and Pelvic Xrays

How would you resuscitate this patient?

Airway with cervical spine protection
• Perform chin lift or jaw thrust
• Clear the airway of foreign bodies

SURGICAL SKILLS

• Insert an oropharyngeal airway
• Establish a definitive airway e.g. intubation or surgical cricothyroidotomy
• Maintain cervical spine in neutral position as necessary when establishing an airway

Breathing
• High flow oxygen via mask reservoir
• Ventilate with bag-mask device
• Intubation

Circulation with haemorhage control
• A least two large bore IV cannula in antecubital fossa and obtain bloods including FBC, lactate and crossmatch
• Pregnancy test for females
• 1 to 2 L bolus of warm IV fluids ie 37 to 40 degrees
• Direct manual pressure for external blood loss from wound
• Tourniquet for massive exsanguination from an extremity, but carry a risk of ischaemic injury and should only be used when direct pressure is not effective
• Management may include chest decompression, pelvic binders, splint application and surgical intervention

What is the secondary survey and when does it start?

The secondary survey does not begin until the primary survey (ABCDEs) is completed, resuscitative efforts are underway and the normalization of vital functions has been demonstrated
The secondary survey is head to toe evaluation of the trauma patient, including a full history and physical examination, including reassessment of all vital signs
Assesses following systems:
o Head and maxillofacial
o Cervical spine and neck
o Chest
o Abdomen
o Perineum, rectum and vagina
o Musculoskeletal
o Neurological

How would you take a history during the ATLS secondary survey?

The **AMPLE** history is a useful mneumonic for this purpose:

• **A**llergies
• **M**edications currently used
• **P**ast illnesses or Pregnancy
• **L**ast meal
• **E**vents or Environment related to the injury

Burns are a specific type of trauma that can be coupled with blunt and penetrating trauma resulting from a burning automobile.

Inhalation injury and carbon monoxide. Therefore it is important to know the circumstances of the burn injury, such as the environment in which the burn injury occurred (open or closed space), the substances consumed by the flames (e.g. plastics and chemicals) and any possible associated injuries which are all factors critical for management.

You have now completed your primary and secondary survey. What do you do next?

- Revaluation – Trauma patients must be constantly revaluated to ensure that new findings are not overlooked and to discover deterioration in previously noted findings.
- Definitive care – Transfer should be considered whenever the patient's treatment need exceeds the capability of the receiving institution

SUMMARY

Assess the multiply injured patient using primary survey (ABCDE) & resuscitation, secondary survey and revaluation. A quick assessment of the A, B and C can be conducted by asking the patient what has happened. An appropriate response suggests there is no major airway compromise, breathing is not compromised and there is no major decrease in level of consciousness. Regardless of the injury, causing airway compression, the first priority is airway management, including clearing the airway, suctioning, administering oxygen and securing the airway. During E, completely undress the patient but prevent hypothermia. Management and adjuncts to primary and secondary surveys can be instituted at the time of assessment. A patients medical history can be taken during the secondary survey using the mnemonic AMPLE, which is critical to identifying injuries. The primary survey should be repeated frequently, and any abnormalities should prompt a thorough reassessment. Early identification of patients requiring transfer to a higher level of care improves outcomes.

TOP TIPS

➕ Don't forget to reevaluate to identify any change in the patient's status that indicates need for additional intervention!

➕ Use your clinical judgement to determine which procedures are necessary, because not all patients require all of these procedures!

➕ Remember 'Blood on the floor + four more'. Chest, pelvis (retroperitoneum), abdomen and thigh.

SURGICAL SKILLS

2.3 | Venepuncture

Scenario

You are the general surgery CT2 on nights. You have been asked by the general surgical registrar to obtain a set of bloods including Liver Function Tests (LFTs), Coagulation & Viral Serology including Hepatitis B, Hepatitis C and HIV on a jaundiced 30-year-old patient with a history of IVDU.

Please proceed to take a set of bloods in this patient.

• Obtain consent for test to be performed. Consent must be obtained for HIV test and the patient has the right to refuse.
• Prepare blood-taking equipment including needle, vacutainer, syringes, blood bottles, sterile wipe, sterile gauze, non-sterile gloves, tourniquet & sharps container
• Choose appropriate blood bottles for task stated
    o Yellow: Liver function tests and viral serology
    o Blue: Coagulation
• Perform hand hygiene using WHO 5 moments for hand hygiene
• Put on well fitting, non sterile gloves
• Disinfect the entry site and allow area to dry
• Do not touch the cleaned site, if it is touched – repeat the disinfection
• Perform venepuncture in the antecubital fossa
• Once sufficient blood has been collected, release the tourniquet before withdrawing the needle
• Withdraw the needle gently and apply gentle pressure to the site with clean gauze
• Fill the laboratory sample tubes
• Draw samples in the correct order to avoid cross-contamination of additives between tubes depending on hospital laboratory guidelines
• Handles sharps safely
    o Dispose of sharps correctly
    o Do not resheath needles
• Match patient to sample and label correctly
• Perform hand hygiene
• Clean up spills

What are the universal precautions in IVDU

Universal precautions refers to the practice, in medicine, of avoiding contact with patient's bodily fluids, by means of wearing non porous articles such as medical gloves, goggles and face shields
• Universal precautions are the infection control techniques that are adopted as if every person treated were infected and therefore precautions are taken to minimize risk
• Includes:
    o Hand hygiene
    o Use of personal protective equipment
    o Safe handling of hypodermic needles and scalpels
    o Aseptic technique

What are the body's defences against bacteria?

- Humoral mechanisms
    - o Innate e.g. complement activation
    - o Acquired e.g. antibody production from plasma cells
- Cell-mediated
    - o Innate e.g. NK cells
    - o Acquired e.g. in relation to bacteria that can grow within human cells such as mycobacteria

What are body's defences against viruses?

- Humoral mechanisms
    - o Antibody production
- Interferon produced by leucocytes and fibroblasts
- Cell mediated e.g. NK cells and cytokines

Why is it important for a surgeon to understand HIV?

- Risk of transmission from infected patient to the surgeon and other staff
- Due to comorbidities and complications at time of surgery
- Nutrition management

What infections are characteristically found in patients with HIV?

- Pneumocystis carinii (pneumocystis jiroveci)
- Herpes zoster and herpes simplex
- Tuberculosis
- Mycobacterium avium intracellular infection (MAI)
- Candidiasis

EXAMINATION SUMMARY

SURGICAL SKILLS

Carry out hand hygiene following the WHO's 5 moments for hand hygiene. Don one pair of non-sterile gloves and use a single-use device for blood sampling and drawing. Disinfect the skin at the venepuncture site and discard the used needle in the sharps bin. Do not overfill or decant a sharps container. Place laboratory sample tubes in a sturdy rack before injecting into the rubber stopper and do not inject it while holding it with the other hand. Do immediately report any incident or accident linked to a needle or sharp injury, and seek assistance. In such an instance, start Post Exposure Prophylaxis to help avert HIV and hepatitis B infections, following hospital protocols.

TOP TIPS

✚ Don't forget to let alcohol or disinfectant dry!

✚ Do not press the syringe plunger to force the blood into a tube, this increases the shear force on red blood cells and increases risk of haemolysis.

2.4 | Cannulation

Scenario

You are the CT2 admitting a patient in the Emergency Department. The 25 year old patient has been admitted with burns following a house fire. On your ABCDE assessment, her vital observations show a heart rate of 120 and a blood pressure of 75 over 50 mmHg.

Please proceed to insert a cannula

Obtain consent for test to be performed. Consent must be obtained for HIV test and the patient has the right to refuse.
• Prepare cannula, saline – 10 ml, syringe – 10 ml, sterile swab, cannula dressing, non-sterile gloves, tourniquet & sharps container
• Apply tourniquet and palpate vein
• Perform hand hygiene using WHO 5 moments for hand hygiene
• Put on well fitting, non sterile gloves
• Disinfect the entry site and allow area to dry
• Do not touch the cleaned site, if it is touched – repeat the disinfection
• Remove cannula sheath, ensure needle's bevel is pointing upwards and insert cannula at 20-40 degrees
• Observe flashback
• Advance the needle a further 1-2mm after flashback to ensure its in the veins lumen
• Withdraw needle slightly and advance cannula into the vein
• Release the tourniquet
• Place some gauze directly underneath the cannula to prevent spills
• Remove the needle
• Place cap on cannula
• Dispose of needle in sharps bin
• Secure the cannula before flushing with 10mls of saline

What is Poiseuille's law?

The rate of flow is proportional to the fourth power of the radius of the cannula and inversely related to its length.

Using this law, deduce and justify which type of cannula or intravenous line would be most suitable for this patient.

Short, large caliber peripheral intravenous lines are preferred for the rapid infusion of large volumes of fluid.

What types of fluids do you know of?

• Colloids
o E.g. Gelofusin, blood
o Natural or synthetic
o Composed of large molecules, generally with molecular weight of >30,000
o Remain within plasma, exerting osmotic pressure
• Crystalloids
o E.g. Normal (0.9% saline or Hartmanns)
o Remain within plasma, exerting osmotic pressure
o In the case of 5% dextrose, once the sugar is metabolized the remaining water extends into the total body compartment

What choice of fluids would you use in an emergency

• Either may be used
• Controversial
• Both are able to provide plasma expansion to support arterial blood pressure in blood loss
• Blood (a colloid) may be required to provide oxygen carrying capacity when tissue oxygenation is affected by loss of red cells
• Crystalloid is not able to provide further oxygen carrying capacity
• Because of the volume of distribution of crystalloid, more is required than colloid to provide a comparable increase in plasma volume

How do you assess the state of hydration clinically

Clinical findings:
      o Skin turgor
      o Capillary refill time
      o Sunken eyes
      o Dry mucous membranes
      o Level of consciousness

• Assess fluid chart for input and output balance
• Tachycardia
• Hypotension
• Measure the central venous pressure (CVP) and determine the respond to a fluid challenge
      o If there is underfilling, the CVP will not increase in response to the challenge

What is the basal water requirement for an adult

30-40ml per kg per day

What are the main fluid compartments of the body and what are their volumes

• Intracellular compartment: 28 L
• Extracellular compartment: 14 L
      o Plasma: 3 L
      o Interstitum: 10L
      o Transcellular: 1L

SUMMARY

Cannulation is an easy station to which you can glean marks. Ensure you have prepared your equipment before commencing the procedure. Disinfect the skin before removing the cannula and always dispose of sharps safely. An understanding of the composition of crystalloid and colloid IV fluids and their components is important.

SURGICAL SKILLS

TOP TIPS

✚ Don't forget to release the tourniquet before removing the needle!

✚ Always dispose of sharps correctly even if distracted by the examiners questions!

2.5 | Central Line

Scenario

You are the vascular CT2 on the ward. You have been asked by the vascular consultant to insert a central venous catheter (CVC) for a patient with peripheral vascular disease who has poor peripheral access and is receiving phlebotoxic antibiotics.

What is Seldinger technique

Seldinger technique is the use of a guidewire to gain safe access to blood vessels and other hollow organs

What are the indications for a central venous catheter?

• Administration of inotropes
• Administration of total parenteral nutrition (TPN)
• Lack of peripheral access
• Central venous pressure (CVP) measurement
• Temporary cardiac pacing
• Haemodialysis

Which vessels can be used for central line insertion?

Internal jugular vein, subclavian vein or femoral vein.

What is the surface anatomy of the internal jugular vein?

The internal jugular vein is located at the apex of the triangle formed by the heads of the sternocleidomastoid muscle and the clavicle.

What is the surface anatomy of the subclavian vein?

The subclavian vein crosses under the clavicle just medial to the midclavicular point.

What imaging is required when inserting a central line?

• Ultrasound (2D) guidance is recommended for CVC in both the elective and emergency situation. It allows precise location of the target vein, anatomical variation and thrombosis within the vein.
• A post-operative CXR is required to exclude iatrogenic pneumothorax.

How would you differentiate the internal jugular vein from the adjacent carotid artery?

• The carotid artery lies medial to the vein in the carotid sheath.
• The artery is smaller, pulsatile and unlike the vein, is not compressible.

Discuss the procedure of inserting a central line

• Gain consent
• Place patient in Trendelenberg position (head down) for internal jugular vein and subclavian vein insertion
• For femoral vein central line insertion, the supine position is adopted
• Identify landmarks and use ultrasound to identify desired vein and adjacent arteries

SURGICAL SKILLS

- Wash hands, don sterile gown and gloves
- Clean the area using appropriate disinfectant, followed by sterile draping
- Apply sterile sheath to ultrasound probe
- Use 1% lignocaine to anaesthetise the area
- Flush all lumens of line with normal saline and then clamp all lumens except Seldinger port
- Advance the needle into internal jugular vein, under ultrasound guidance until flashback of blood is visualized
- Remove syringe and immediately insert Seldinger wire
- Keeping hold of Seldinger wire, remove needle whilst ensuring wire stays in the vein
- Pass the dilator over the wire and gently but firmly dilate a tract through to the internal jugular vein
- Remove the dilator and pass the central line over the seldinger wire
- Once the central line is in place, remove the wire
- Aspirate and flush all lumens, then reclamp and apply lumen caps
- Secure the catheter using sutures and apply a clear dressing
- Attach central line to pressure bag to allow CVP monitoring
- Obtain a CXR to exclude iatrogenic pneumothorax
- Clear documentation of date of insertion and monitor for infection

What are the complications of central line insertion?

- Pneumothorax
- Haemothorax
- Arterial injury
- Air embolism
- Haemorrhage
- Haematoma
- Line sepsis
- Line blockage
- Arrhythmia

What is Central Venous Pressure, what is the normal value and what does it indicate?

- The Central Venous Pressure is expressed in cmH20 above a point level with the right atrium.
- The normal value is 0-8cm H_2O
- It gives a useful indication of filling status and right ventricular preload

What are causes of an increased and decreased CVP?

- Increased CVP:
  - o Increased intra-thoracic pressure
  - o Impaired cardiac function e.g. congestive heart failure or cardiac tamponade
  - o Hypervolaemia
  - o Superior Vena Cava (SVC) obstruction
- Decreased CVP:
  - o Hypovolaemia
  - o Reduced intrathoracic pressure e.g inspiration

What are contraindications to central line insertion?

- Coagulopathy
- Local infection
- Patient non-compliance

SUMMARY

Central lines are inserted for a number of reasons including haemodynamic monitoring, IV delivery of blood products and drugs, haemodialysis, TPN & management of perioperative fluids. Central venous access is achieved by puncturing a central vein and using Seldinger technique to pass the line into the relevant vein. Knowledge of the expected anatomical relationship of the vein to its comparable artery is key and ultrasound guidance is recommended. Commonly used veins are the internal jugular vein, subclavian vein and the femoral vein. Frequently encountered complications are pneumothorax, arterial puncture and haemorrhage, which delay treatment.

TOP TIPS

➕ A thorough understanding of the anatomy of the neck will help for internal jugular vein catheterization!

➕ Never let go of the Seldinger wire!

SURGICAL SKILLS

2.6 | Chest Drain

Scenario

A 32-year-old man has fallen off his motorbike at a speed of 30mph. He is brought into the accident and emergency department by paramedics.

How would you approach this patient?

I would take an ABCDE approach to the management of this patient.

A: Airway with c-spine control
• I would start by talking to patient, whilst ensuring that the cervical spine was immobilized with a hard collar, blocks and tape (i.e. immobilisation with three-point fixation).
• "Talking patients" who make appropriate verbal response, provide reassurance that the airway is patent, ventilation is intact, and brain perfusion is adequate.
• I would also apply 15 litres of oxygen via a non-rebreathe mask.

B: Breathing
• I would measure respiratory rate, observe accessory muscle use and monitor oxygen saturation.
• I would look and feel for chest expansion, and assess whether it is equal bilaterally.
• On lung percussion, I would assess for any dullness, suggestive of a haemothorax or hyper-resonance, suggestive of a pneumothorax.
• I would assess whether the trachea was central or deviated.
• On auscultate of both lungs, I would look for any reduced air entry or added sounds.

Findings

His respiratory rate is 28 breaths per minute and SO2 92% on 15L of oxygen. He has reduced air entry on the right side with hyperresonance on percussion and the trachea is deviated to the left.

Given the above clinical findings, what are you concerned about?

A right-sided tension pneumothorax.

Describe the immediate management and anatomical landmarks.

This patient requires immediate needle decompression of his tension pneumothorax. I would obtain verbal consent and position the patient at 45 degrees. I would palpate for the second intercostal space midclavicular line and use a large bore (size 16-18 gauge) cannula to decompress the pneumothorax. In the meantime, I would ask for a chest drain kit to be prepared.

The patient makes some improvement. You continue with your primary survey and the nurse tells you that his oxygen saturations are dropping again. What would you do?

I would go back to reassess 'A' (the airway) and ensure that it is still patent, followed by reassessment of 'B' (breathing). At this stage, it is likely that the patient requires insertion of a surgical chest drain as definitive management of his pneumothorax, before moving on to an assessment of his circulation.

What is the 'safe zone'?

This is the area of safety for inserting a chest drain, as described by the British Thoracic Society (see diagram below). More specifically, the tube is inserted into the 5th intercostal space slightly anterior to the mid axillary line.

The Boundaries are:
* Lateral border of pectoralis major
* Anterior border of latissimus dorsi
* 5th intercostal space; a horizontal line superior to the nipple
* A horizontal line inferior to the axilla

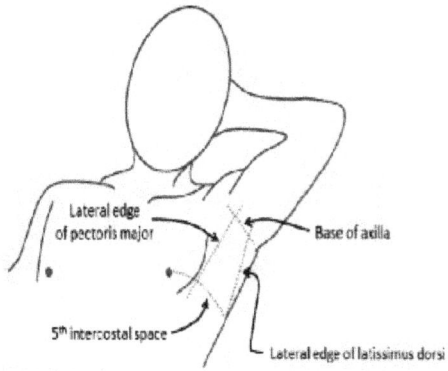

Lateral edge of pectoris major — Base of axilla

5th intercostal space

Lateral edge of latissimus dorsi

Show me how you would insert a chest drain in this patient.

• **Step 1:** In a conscious patient, I would explain the procedure and obtain verbal consent. I would also check for any allergies.
• **Step 2:** Position the patient at 45 degrees, with their right hand behind their head. Prepare and sterile drape the site of chest tube insertion.
• **Step 3:** Apply local anaesthetic to include the periosteum and the pleura at the point of incision in the triangle of safety.
• **Step 4:** Make a 2cm transverse skin incision. Sharp dissect through the subcutaneous tissue to ABOVE the rib.
• **Step 5:** Blunt dissect, using artery forceps, through the intercostal muscles in an oblique plane.
• **Step 6:** Blunt dissect the parietal pleura.
• **Step 7:** Using a finger sweep along the tract into the intrapleural space.
• **Step 8:** Remove the central trocar of the chest drain, and aim and place the chest drain at the apex of the chest.
• **Step 9:** Secure the chest tube to the skin with a purse string 1/0 silk suture and adhesive dressing.
• **Step 10:** Connect the chest tube to an underwater seal chest drain bottle.

What would you do once you have completed chest drain insertion?

• I would ensure that the chest drain is working by observing air swinging in the tube and air bubbles in the underwater seal bottle.
• I would request an erect CXR to check for resolution of the pneumothorax and correct chest drain placement.
• Following this intervention, I would go back and re-assess patient (ABCDE).

SURGICAL SKILLS

You are presented with two plain radiographs. Describe what you can see?

You should answer this question systematically. Start with the statement " This is a plain erect anteroposterior chest radiograph of Mr James taken on the 15th of November 2015 at 15:30hrs".

Usually in these scenarios, you will not be expected to go through the description of the x-ray in its entirety. The examiner will usually ask you to identify the most obvious abnormality and the diagnosis, with subsequent discussion relating to the management of the pathology.

> ⌒ **Findings**
>
> **Chest X-Ray 1:** There is an evidence of a right-sided tension pneumothorax supported by the absence of lung markings, evident lung edges, mediastinal shift and tracheal deviation to the left.

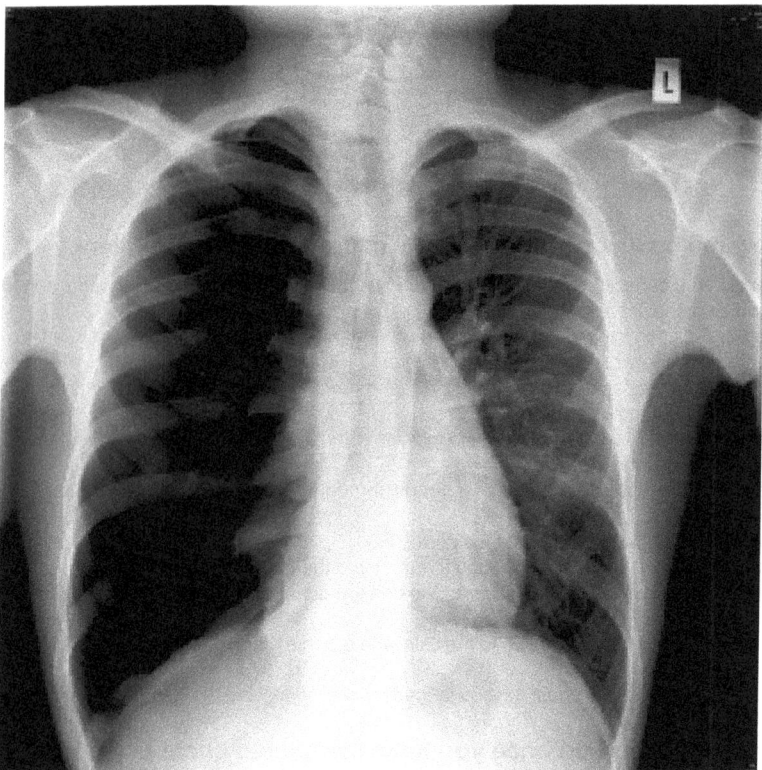

> ⌒ **Findings**
>
> **Chest X-Ray 2:** The second chest x-ray shows incomplete resolution of the tension pneumothorax with evidence an unsatisfactory chest tube position.

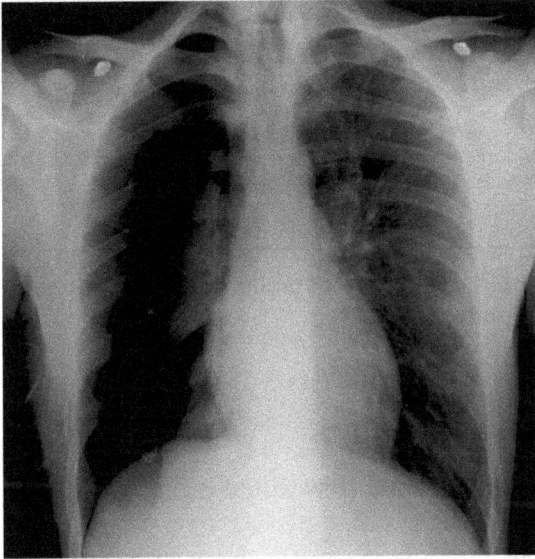

SUMMARY

Chest Drain Insertion

• **Step 1:** In a conscious patient, I would explain the procedure and obtain verbal consent. I would also check for any allergies.
• **Step 2:** Position the patient at 45 degrees, with their right hand behind their head. Prepare and sterile drape the site of chest tube insertion.
• **Step 3:** Apply local anaesthetic to include the periosteum and the pleura at the point of incision in the triangle of safety.
• **Step 4:** Make a 2cm transverse skin incision. Sharp dissect through the subcutaneous tissue to ABOVE the rib.
• **Step 5:** Blunt dissect, using artery forceps, through the intercostal muscles in an oblique plane.
• **Step 6:** Blunt dissect the parietal pleura.
• **Step 7:** Using a finger sweep along the tract into the intrapleural space.
• **Step 8:** Remove the central trocar of the chest drain, and aim and place the chest drain at the apex of the chest.
• **Step 9:** Secure the chest tube to the skin with a purse string 1/0 silk suture and adhesive dressing.
• **Step 10:** Connect the chest tube to an underwater seal chest drain bottle.

TOP TIPS

You may find clues telling you that this is a chest drain station. However, you should answer questions systematically and you will be directed appropriately.

SURGICAL SKILLS

2.7 | Wound Debridement

Scenario

You are the vascular registrar on call and you are called by the A&E SHO to see a 52 year old farmer who has sustained a deep wound to his forearm whilst cutting timber in his farm.

What else would you like to establish over the phone to help you prioritise the patient?

Is there:
- Evidence of neurovascular injury?
- Associated bony injury?
- Other significant injuries?

You go to see the patient. How would you approach his management?

I would take an ABCDE approach to the management of this patient. Once I have assessed his airway, cervical spine and breathing, I would assess his circulation. At this point I would also review the wound to ensure that there is no active or uncontrolled haemorrhage.

What haemorrhage control options are you aware of?

- Non-surgical
  - o Direct pressure
  - o Tourniquet
- Surgical/Interventional
  - o Ligation of bleeding vessels
  - o Diathermy
  - o Embolisation

You remove the dressings in order to examine the wound. Describe how you would do that.

I will explain to the patient what I am about to do and obtain verbal consent. I will ask about pain and give adequate analgesia. I would remove the dressing and inspect the wound. Using the departmental camera, I would take a photograph of the wound for documentation.

> ### 👓 Findings
>
> There is an approximately 5cm X 2cm longitudinal, traumatic laceration overlying the flexor aspect of the mid-third of the right forearm. The wound edges are partially devitalised. There is evidence of dirt and gravel contamination. The wound is deep. This wound requires exploration under general anaesthesia.

What would you do next?

- Rinse the wound with 250mls of normal saline and cover with a sterile, non-adhesive

dressing gauze.
• Administer antibiotics, as per local hospital protocol.
• As the wound is heavily contaminated, you should be concerned about tetanus. Therefore, prescribe a tetanus booster/immunoglobulins, if the patient is not fully immunized.
• Order a plain x-ray of the limb to rule out any underlying fracture and/or radio-opaque foreign bodies e.g. glass.
• Consent the patient and mark the limb with an arrow.
• Keep the patient NBM and inform theatre staff and the anaesthetist.

You have discussed the case with your consultant who is happy for you to take the patient for wound washout and debridement. The patient is in theatre. Show me how you would perform the procedure.

- Perform the WHO theatre checklist.
- Administer antibiotics, as per trust protocol.
- Position the patient supine position with the arm out on an arm table.
- Scrub, prepare and drape the arm.
- Start by examining the wound using toothed forceps to raise the skin edges and non-toothed forceps to pick up any foreign bodies.
- Do not put your hand blindly into the wound.
- Systematically explore the wound from from proximal to distal and from superficial to deep.
- Ask your assistant to hold a kidney bowl underneath the arm to collect irrigation fluid and gently irrigate the wound to facilitate vision.
- Check for bleeding and evidence of damage to muscles, tendons, nerves or vessels.
- Debride any unhealthy tissue using a scalpel or scissor.
- Ensure haemostasis throughout the procedure.
- Once satisfied with the exploration, irrigate the wound thoroughly with a litre of warmed saline.
- If wound is heavily contaminated, pack the wound with non-adhesive packing and plan for either a delayed primary closure or healing by secondary intention.
- Apply blue gauze and wrap the forearm with wool and crepe.

What post-operative instructions would you document in the operative notes?

• Elevate the arm in a sling to help alleviate any arm swelling
• Regularly assess neurovascular status of the limb
• Continue with IV antibiotics for 24 hours
• Ensure adequate analgesia is prescribed and given.

What types of wound healing do you know of?

• Healing by primary intention – wound edges are approximated immediately e.g. in clean wounds.
• Healing by secondary intention – the wound is not closed. This may be because of the contamination e.g. an abscess cavity
• Healing by delayed primary intention e.g. fasciotomies for compartment syndrome.

What types of injuries are you aware of?

• Non-Penetrating e.g. blunt trauma
• Penetrating e.g. stab wounds, gunshot wounds

SURGICAL SKILLS

Why is it important to document the nature of the wound?

• Forensic evidence.
• For transmission of information to colleagues.
• An understanding of the size, site, depth and affected structures will help guide further management.

What would you do if you have discovered an associated displaced ulna fracture with this patient's injury?

I would liaise with the trauma and orthopaedics team. This patient will require washout, debridement and application of an external fixator.

Which other teams would you potentially need to liaise with?

• Plastic surgeons, as patient might require skin grafting and there may also be an associated tendon or nerve injury.
• Vascular surgeons, if there is an associated arterial injury.

SUMMARY

Contaminated wounds need to be washed and debrided to avoid infection. With any open laceration care should be taken to identify associated injuries and handle tissue with care.

The wound should be careful inspected and documented and antibiotics and tetanus updates provided as required. Underlying injuries such as open fractures or soft-tissue injuries should be looked for and the wound should be lightly covered and the patient kept nil by mouth pending formal washout.

TOP TIPS

➕ Speak to the patient in this scenario and explain to them what you are about to do if they are awake i.e. do not ignore the patient.

➕ If the scenario tells you that your consultant has been called away, you need to start by checking the consent form, side of procedure and indication for the operation before continuing.

2.8 Discharge Summary

Scenario

You are the general surgical SHO in a district general hospital. A 75 years old male was admitted over the weekend for management of his necrotic toe. He starts complaining of central abdominal pain. He has a significant vascular history. You suspect a ruptured AAA and arrange for a contrast enhanced CT angiogram. You are aware that there are no vascular services are available at your hospital. Your consultant arranges for transfer to another hospital and asks you to write a discharge/transfer letter.

Describe what you would write in your discharge/transfer letter.

1. Hospital Name
2. Patient Identifiers
   - Full Name
   - Hospital number
   - NHS number
   - Date of birth
   - Address and post code
4. GP ID
   - Name
   - GP practice name
   - Address
5. Consultant in charge
   - Full name
   - Speciality
   - Contact details
6. Ward/Department
7. Contact details (phone number)
8. Date of admission
9. Date of discharge
10. Primary discharge diagnosis (Confirmed/provisional)
11. Secondary discharge diagnosis
12. Presenting complaint
13. Mode of admission
14. Source of referral
15. Significant operations/procedures
16. Clinical Progress
    - Investigations
    - Complications
    - Relevant information
17. Results awaited
18. Investigations pending
19. Allergies (Specify name of allergen and type of reaction)
20. Medicines stopped on discharge
21. New medicines started during admission
22. Continuing medicines on discharge
    - Name of medicine
    - Formulation
    - Route

- Frequency
- Duration of treatment
- Number of days supply

23. **Follow up arrangements**
24. **Copies**
    - To pharmacy/patient/carer
25. **Specify if extended document to follow**
26. **Consultant sign off and comment**
27. **Signature, name and position of person writing the summary**

SUMMARY

This station often leaves the candidate alone with a set of notes and limited time to write the discharge summary. The key is to skim through the notes and quickly identify the salient points. Then note down the key components of the discharge summary as outlined above in a logical sequence.

TOP TIPS

✚ The station can be tight for time, do not panic and stick to a logical sequence when writing the discharge summary.

✚ Don't forget simple things like dating and signing

2.9 | Fine Needle Aspiration

Scenario

You are attending the breast clinic with your team. You have seen a 58 years old lady with a breast lump. Your consultant advises you to perform a FNA and prepare the slides. He asks you a number of questions.

What other types of biopsy methods are you aware of?

- Punch Biopsy
- Core Biopsy
- Surgical Biopsy
- Washings, scrapes and brushings.

Show me how you would perform a FNA of a palpable breast lump.

State that you would gain informed consent. Check the side of the procedure and ask for a chaperone to be present.
- **Step 1:** Prepare the necessary equipment (slides, needle and syringe)
- **Step 2:** Number the slides and put the patients name on each slide.
- **Step 3:** Wash your hands and wear sterile gloves. Clean the skin using chlorhexadine.
- **Step 4:** Whilst holding the lump between two fingers, puncture the skin overlying the lump with a small gauge needle (23-27 Gauge) at a 30-45 degrees angle and pull the plunger of the syringe back to create a negative pressure.
- **Step 3:** Move the needle back and forth, and in a circular motion until you see fluid being aspirated. Withdraw the needle.
- **Step 4:** Apply a small dressing to the needle puncture site.
- **Step 5:** Place the specimen (one or two drops) on the slides labelled numbers 1 to 3 (in that order).
- **Step 6:** If there is only a small amount of aspirate, express some of the specimen within the needle by applying positive pressure using the syringe.
- **Step 7:** Apply glass onto each slide. Complete the histopathology form and send this with the specimen to the lab.
- **Step 8:** Dispose of sharps carefully and wash your hands.

Can you list 4 advantages and 2 disadvantages of FNA?

- Advantages:
  - o Less invasive
  - o Fast
  - o Cheap
  - o Results are easily interpreted.

- Disadvantages:
  - o Cannot assess tissue architecture
  - o High rate of false negative results in inexperienced hands.

Can you list other parts of body other than the breast where FNA has a role?

- Thyroid
- Superficial lymph nodes
- Mediastinum (e.g. ultrasound-guided transbronchial FNA for mediastinal masses)

SURGICAL SKILLS

• Deeper Structure such as the liver, pancreas, kidney and lungs (usually ultrasound or CT guided)

Can you list 8 microscopic features of malignancy?

• Invasion
• Architectural abnormalities
• Necrosis
• Nuclear abnormalities: pleomorphism, enlargement, dense chromatin and chromatin clumping.
• Increased nuclear/cytoplasmic ratio.
• Irregular Mitoses.
• Lack of differentiation.

What is the most significant factor which distinguishes tumour in-situ from malignancy?

Invasion of the basement membrane.

What is the difference between histology and cytology?

Cytology looks at the characteristics of cells only; histology looks at the cells within its local tissue architecture.

Can you list the pros and cons of histological sampling, for example, core biopsy?

• Pros:
          o Gives information on tissue architecture and invasion, so it is useful in tumour staging.
• Cons:
          o Takes longer to report as it requires fixation and processing
          o More expensive
          o More invasive than cytology
          o Can be distressing to the patient
          o Potential of spreading of tumour cells (seeding).

What is the difference between Staging and Grading?

Staging is the extent to which the cancer has developed by spreading. Grading is how well the tumour is differentiated based on its histological architecture, i.e. the extent to which the tumour resembles normal tissue architecture.

Can you name some staging systems used in oncology?

• TNM (Tumour, Nodes, Metastasis) scoring system
• Breslow's thickness (used for skin cancer)
• Duke's staging system (used for colorectal cancer)

What are the most important factors affecting prognosis?

• Stage of the tumour (more important than grade) and grade of the tumour.
• Poorly differentiated tumours, evidence of perivascular and/or perineural invasion and positive resection margin are all associated with a poor prognosis.

What do you understand by the term Tumour Marker?

A tumour marker is a substance that can be found to be elevated in the blood, urine or body tissues of a patient with cancer. It is either produced directly by the tumour or by non-tumour cells in response to the tumour. It can be used to for:
• Screening for common cancers
• Aiding diagnosis
• Monitoring the response to treatment and for recurrence.

Can you give 4 examples and the tumour associated with each?

• CEA (Carcinoembryonic Antigen) - Colorectal Cancer
• CA125 (Cancer antigen 125) - Ovarian Cancer
• CA19-9 (Cancer antigen 19-9) - Pancreatic Cancer
• PSA (Prostate-Specific Antigen) - Prostate Cancer
• AFP (Alpha Fetoprotein) - Hepatocellular Cancer and Non-Seminoma Testicular Cancer

SUMMARY

State that you would gain informed consent. Check the side of the procedure and ask for a chaperone to be present.

• **Step 1:** Prepare the necessary equipment (slides, needle and syringe)
• **Step 2:** Number the slides and put the patients name on each slide.
• **Step 3:** Wash your hands and wear sterile gloves. Clean the skin using chlorhexadine.
• **Step 4:** Whilst holding the lump between two fingers, puncture the skin overlying the lump with a small gauge needle (23-27 Gauge) at a 30-45 degrees angle and pull the plunger of the syringe back to create a negative pressure.
• **Step 3:** Move the needle back and forth, and in a circular motion until you see fluid being aspirated. Withdraw the needle.
• **Step 4:** Apply a small dressing to the needle puncture site.
• **Step 5:** Place the specimen (one or two drops) on the slides labelled numbers 1 to 3 (in that order).
• **Step 6:** If there is only a small amount of aspirate, express some of the specimen within the needle by applying positive pressure using the syringe.
• **Step 7:** Apply glass onto each slide. Complete the histopathology form and send this with the specimen to the lab.
• **Step 8:** Dispose of sharps carefully and wash your hands.

TOP TIPS

Usually actors/actresses will be acting worried and you will be assessed on how you respond to this, be professional and reassuring.

SURGICAL SKILLS

2.10 Joint Aspiration

Scenario

You are the orthopaedic SHO on call. A&E is busy and the nurse in charge calls and asks you to kindly see a 60-year-old insulin dependent diabetic who has a painful swollen knee.

What are the key points you will be looking for in the history and examination?

History:
- Pain: Onset, duration, site, character, radiation and history of associated trauma
- Mobility: range of movement, ability to weight bear, history of the joint giving way
- Swelling: Onset, duration and deterioration versus improvement of swelling
- Systematic enquiry: Involvement of other joints, fevers.
- Past Medical History:
   o Previous injuries, previous episodes, history of surgery to the knee.
   o Evidence of immunsupression, e.g. diabetes mellitus, chronic kidney disease, steroids use.
- Medications: Diuretics, Immunosuppressants, Aspirin.

Examination (Look, Feel and Move):
- Skin Colour
- Scars
- Effusion size
- Deformities
- Temperature
- Tenderness
- Range of movement
- Joint Stability
- Examination of the hip and ankle and any other affected joints

Give 3 possible causes of the knee swelling:

- Bone/soft tissue injury
- Septic Arthritis
- Gout
- Pseudogout

What investigations will you order for this patient?

- Bloods tests: FBC, U&E, CRP, ESR
- Imaging: weight bearing AP, lateral and skyline plain films of both knees.
- Knee aspiration

Show me how you would aspirate this gentleman's knee

- Obtain informed consent
- Lie the patient at 30 degrees
- Prepare your equipment
- Wash your hands
- Prep and drape the knee in the standard manner
- Wearing sterile gloves, palpate the patella
- Penetrate the patella at the lateral aspect of its upper pole using a large bore needle

(white) and aiming at 30 degrees towards the joint line. NB: A large bore needle is less likely to be blocked by pus.
• Once you see a flashback of fluid, start aspirating.
• Leave the needle in situ and exchange the syringe if needed, to aspirate the maximum amount of fluid possible.
• Make a comment on the appearance of the aspirated fluid
• Withdraw the needle and syringe and apply an adhesive small dressing over the puncture site
• Label the specimen and complete the request form
• Thank the patient and wash your hands.

What tests would you do on the knee aspirate?

• White cell count and differential
• Gram stain and culture
• Polarizing light microscopy

If you suspect this patient has Gout what will you be expecting to see on light microscopy?

Monosodium urate crystals (birefringent crystals).

What are the most likely causative organisms of septic arthritis?

• Staphylococcus sp is the most common cause.
• Streptococcus sp and Neisseria gonorrhoea is common in patients with splenic dysfunction
• Gram-negative bacteria, fungal species and Mycoplasma hominis are common in immunocompromised patients.

Can you mention 5 risk factors for Septic Arthritis?

• Extremes of age
• Immunosuppression
• Intravenous drug abuse
• Central venous line
• Prosthetic Joint
• Joint Instrumentation
• Bacteraemia

What are the risk factors for gout?

• Non-modifiable:
    o Age
    o Gender (male>female)
    o Race
• Modifiable:
    o Hyperuricaemia
    o Obesity
    o Hypertension
    o Hyperlipidaemia
    o Diabetes mellitus
    o Alcohol
    o Chronic kidney disease.

Can you name any medications implemented in gout?

SURGICAL SKILLS

Mnemonic: **CANT LEAP**
- **C**yclophosaphimde
- **A**spirin
- **N**icotine
- **T**hiazide
- **L**oop Duretic
- **E**thambutamol
- **A**lcohol
- **P**yrazinamide.

What is the difference between gout and pseudogout?

Gout is caused by hyperuricemia and leads to crystalline monosodium urate (uric acid) deposition in the blood and joint fluid. In pseudogout there is abnormal calcium pyrophosphate deposition in the joint cartilage and fluid (chondrocalcinosis).

What is the antibiotic of choice for treatment in septic arthritis?

The initial choice of antibiotic depends hospital guidelines and on the most likely causative organism based on gram stain results and the clinical presentation. If the causative organism is a gram positive organism, then vancomycin is usually given as a first-line. If it is a gram-negative organism, then third generation cephalosporins, such as, ceftriaxone or cefotaxime should be considered.

Apart from medical management of septic arthritis, are there any other treatment options implicated?

Prompt surgical drainage in the form of open surgical washout is important to prevent further damage to the joint.

If this patient had a total knee replacement 5 years ago and you suspect that the implant is infected, what do you do?

Having taken history, examined the patient and ordered the appropriate investigations, the next step would be to inform my senior collegaues and arrange for this patient to have an aspiration/washout of the knee joint in theatre.
Depending on the blood tests and microbiology results, a decision will need to be made regarding whether the prosthetic joint can salvaged or whether a revision operation is required. The type of antibiotic and duration of therapy will also need to be considered.

SUMMARY

Knee Joint Aspiration
- Obtain informed consent
- Lie the patient at 30 degrees
- Prepare your equipment
- Wash your hands
- Prep and drape the knee in the standard manner
- Wearing sterile gloves, palpate the patella
- Penetrate the patella at the lateral aspect of its upper pole using a large bore needle (white) and aiming at 30 degrees towards the joint line. NB: A large bore needle is less likely to be blocked by pus.
- Once you see a flashback of fluid, start aspirating.
- Leave the needle in situ and exchange the syringe if needed, to aspirate the maximum

amount of fluid possible.
• Make a comment on the appearance of the aspirated fluid
• Withdraw the needle and syringe and apply an adhesive small dressing over the puncture site
• Label the specimen and complete the request form
• Thank the patient and wash your hands.

TOP TIPS

➕ Knee swelling and pain in a prosthetic knee should be considered infective in aetiology until proven otherwise.

➕ Tissue sampling is crucial before commencing antibiotics, unless the patient is septic.

➕ Check INR before aspirating patients who are on warfarin to avoid significant haemarthrosis.

SURGICAL SKILLS

2.11 | Knot Tying

Scenario

You are assisting your consultant in an open nephrectomy and he asks you to tie off the renal artery using a single-handed reef knot. There are a range of different suture packs available including mersilk, ethilon, vicryl, plain, PDS, prolene and monocryl. Your consultant asks you to use a braided absorbable suture

Perform a single handed reef knot with a braided absorbable suture.

The first step is to select the appropriate suture which in this case is vicryl.
A reef knot is made up of 2 throws;
• The first throw starts by holding the short end of suture between the thumb and fourth finger of your non dominant hand with the palm facing upwards (step 1).
• The long end is picked up and laid over the non-dominant index and middle fingers (step 2).
• Flex the non-dominant middle finger so that the suture lies behind the middle finger (step 3).
• Release the short end and pull it through with your non-dominant hand (Step 4)

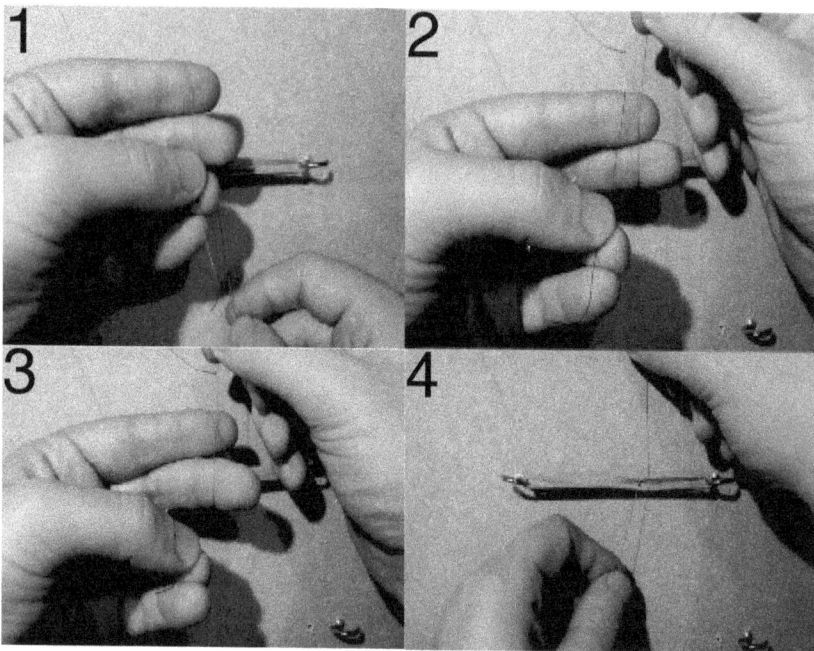

The second throw continues without releasing the suture ends
• The non-dominant hand is turned palm upwards and the suture lies over the middle, fourth and fifth fingers (Step 5).
• The long end is laid parallel to the short end on the middle, fourth and fifth fingers (Step 6).
• The middle finger is flexed so that the suture lies behind the middle finger (Step 7)
• The suture is pulled through to create a square knot (Step 8)

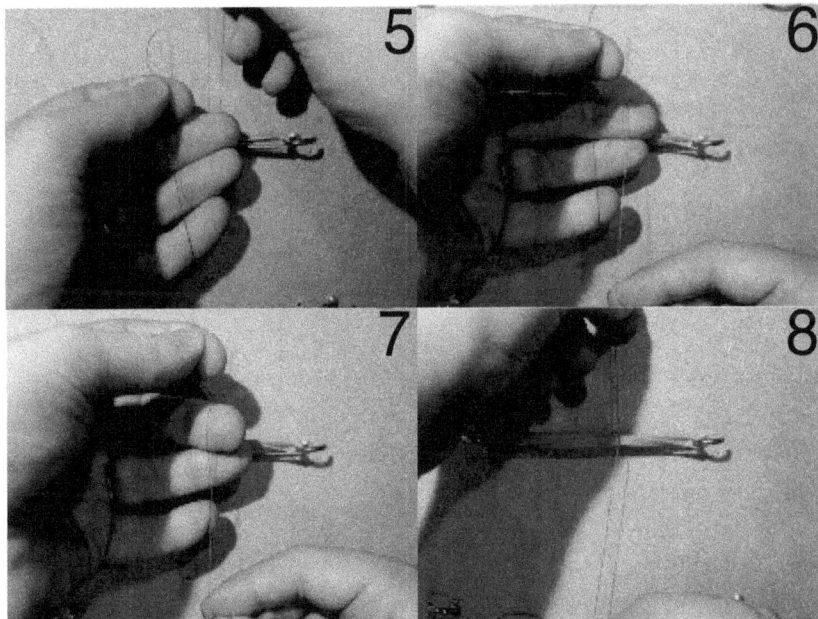

How many throws would you complete for this suture and why

Three throws as it is a braded suture

What is Vicryl made of?

Polyglactin 910

How many days does Vicryl retain its tensile strength for?

Vicryl retains 50% of its tensile at 3 weeks and 25% of its tensile strength at 4 weeks. It is fully absorbed by approximately 2 months

Name two absorbable monofilament sutures

Monocryl and PDS

Name two non-absorbable monofilament sutures

Prolene and Ethilon

Name one non-absorbable braided sutures

Silk

SURGICAL SKILLS

Name an additional knot other than a reef knot

A surgeon's knot

What types of needles do you know?

Needs can be classified by shape or type
i. Shape: Straight, circle, curved or J shaped
ii. Point:

  a. Cutting needle: Has a very sharp tip and sharp edges so it passes easily through tissue. Cutting needles are mainly used for skin sutures
  b. Tapered (or round bodied) needles: Have a sharp tip and smooth edges so are used for deeper tissues (bloods vessels etc.)
  c. Blunt: A blunt point and used to suture friable tissues and vascular organs such as kidney and livers

SUMMARY

This station tests both your knowledge of types of sutures and your knot tying skills. The first stage is selecting the correct suture and then tying a fluent, square knot.

TOP TIPS

➕ Learn the properties of each suture so that you can easily select 'a braided absorbable suture', 'a monofilament absorbable suture', 'a braded non-absorbable suture' or 'monofilament non-absorbable suture'

➕ Practice your knot tying focusing on technique rather than speed. It is more important that you have square knots than a very fast technique

2.12 | Local Anaesthetic

Scenario

A 45 year old woman has been listed for excision of a benign naevus under local anaesthetic. Please demonstrate how to infiltrate 1% lidocaine for the procedure.

Describe what you do before infiltrating the local anesthetic?

Start by introducing yourself and checking the patient, consent form and explaining the procedure

i. Introduce yourself
ii. Patient checks
  • Confirm the patients' name and date of birth
  • Check if they are on any medications, especially anticoagulants, and their allergy status
  • Check if they have a recent documented weight for safe dosing of the local anaesthetic
iii. Consent form
  • Check the consent form and that it is signed and dated by the patient and surgeon
  • Explain the procedure including that they will feel a sharp scratch and burning sensation from the lidocaine
  •

What equipment will you need for to use to infiltrate local anesthetic ?

The following equipment will be needed
i. Alcohol swab
ii. 21G (Green) needle
iii. 10ml syringe
iv. 1% lidocaine
v. 25G (orange) needle
vi.

How would you perform the procedure?

i. Check local anaesthetic
  • Confirm the dose and expiry date of the lidocaine with the examiner
ii. Draw up local anaesthetic with a 21G needle
  • You can ask the examiner for assistance holding the bottle while you draw it up
iii. Clean skin with alcohol swab
iv. Warn the patient they will feel a sharp scratch
v. Pull back on the syringe prior to starting to infiltrate to check you are not in a blood vessel
vi. Infiltrate slowly around the lesion so until you have encircled the lesion
vii.

How would you complete the procedure

i. Wait at least 5 minutes before checking efficacy
ii. Check efficacy using toothed forceps and asking if the patient can feel it
iii. Document dosage in notes

What category of local anaesthetic lidocaine? What other types of local anaesthetic do you know?

- Local anaesthetics can be split into two categories
  i. Amides: Lidocaine and bupivacaine
  ii. Esters: Procaine and cocaine

What is the onset of action of lidocaine and bupivacaine

- Lidocaine has a rapid onset of action within 2 to 5 minutes of injection
- Bupivicaine has a slower onset of action within 5 to 10 minutes after injection

What is the duration of effect of lidocaine and bupivacaine

- Lidocaine has a shorter duration of action of approximately 1 to 2 hours (3 hours with adrenaline)
- Bupivicaine has a longer duration of action of approximately 4 to 8 hours

Why would you use lidocaine with adrenaline

- The addition of adrenaline causes local vasoconstriction which
  i. Prolongs the effect of lidocaine by reducing systemic absorption
  ii. Decreases bleeding

Where is lidocaine with adrenaline contraindicated

- In areas supplied by end arteries including fingers, toes, nose and penis

What is the maximum safe dose of lidocaine with and without adrenaline

- Without adrenaline: 3mg / kg
- With adrenaline: 7mg/kg

What is the maximum safe dose of bupivacaine

- 2mg/kg

Calculate the maximum safe dose of 1% lidocaine without adrenaline which can be administered to 50kg woman

- Maximum safe dose = 3mg/kg x 50kg
  = 150mg
  – 1% lidocaine has 10ml per ml
- 150mg / 10 mg per ml = 15ml

What are the signs and symptoms of lidocaine toxicity

- There are a range of symptoms related to the degree of toxicity
  - Early symptoms: Tinnitus, perioral paresthesia and metal taste in mouse
  - Late symptoms: Bradycardia, reduced GCS and respiratory depression

How would you treat lidocaine toxicity

- Immediately stop lidocaine administration
- Administer lipid emulsion (Intralipid 20%) at 1.5ml/Kg over 1 minute as a bolus

EXAMINATION SUMMARY

Wash Your Hands
Ensure that you are seen by the examiners to wash your hands using alcohol gel provided.

Introduce, Explain and perform safety checks of patient and consent form
Start by introducing yourself and explaining the procedure. Then perform the essential safety checks of the patient and the consent form

Prepare equipment and Check local anaesthetic
Check that you have all your equipment available and check the strength and expiry date of the local anaesthetic

Draw up and administer local anaesthetic
Draw up with a 21G needle and administer with a 25G needle. Always withdraw the syringe before starting to administer the local anaesthetic

Check efficacy
Offer to wait 5 minutes before testing efficacy

TOP TIPS

➕ The administration of local anaesthetic is relatively simple. The key is that you show all the safety aspects including checking the consent form, expiry date of local anaesthetic and withdrawing the syringe prior to infiltrating the local anaesthetic

➕ It is essential that you know the maximum safe doses of both lidocaine and bupivacaine and the symptoms of toxicity

SURGICAL SKILLS

2.13 | Lumbar Puncture

Scenario

A 47 year old woman presents with a sudden onset generalised headache, neck pain and vomiting. She has a past medical history of poorly controlled hypertension. On examination she has a positive Kernig's and Brudxzinski's sign. A non-contrast CT head did not identify any evidence of subarachnoid haemorrhage. You are on-call for the neurosurgical department and are asked to perform a lumbar puncture to exclude a subarachnoid haemorrhage. Please perform this procedure.

Describe what you do before starting the procedure

Start by introducing yourself and checking the patient, consent form and explaining the procedure

i. Introduce yourself
ii. Patient checks
   • Confirm the patients' name and date of birth
   • Check if they are on any medications, especially anticoagulants, and their allergy status
   • Request to review the CT head looking for any signs of raised ICP
iii. Consent form
   • Check the consent form and that it is signed and dated
   • Explain the procedure including that a needle will be inserted into her back after giving local anaesthetic
   • Explain the risks including a post lumbar puncture headaches, pain at insertion site, bleeding and infection.

What equipment will you need for the procedure?

The following equipment will be needed
i.   Sterile gown and gloves
ii. Marker pen
iii. Local anaesthetic (e.g. 1% lidocaine)
iv. Skin preparation (e.g. chlorhexidine 2%)
v.   Needles 21G and 25G
vi. Syringe
vii. Spinal needle
viii. Manometer
ix. Xanthochromia bottle
x.   Specimen bottles labelled 1,2,3,4

How would you position the patient and identify the landmarks for insertion

i. Position the patient either sitting or in the left lateral decubitus position
   • It is generally easier to perform LPs with the patient sitting up but the opening pressure cannot be accurately measured in this position
ii. Identify insertion site
   • Identify the insertion site and palpate the patients' anterior superior iliac spine and draw a line between them (Tuffier's line). This corresponds to approximately level of L4

- Palpate the vertebral process of L4 and identify the vertebral space above (L3/L4) and below (L4/L5)

Demonstrate how you would perform the procedure

i. Clean and drape
   - Prepare the skin with chlorhexidine 2%
   - Drape the patient using an aseptic technique
ii. Local anaesthetic
   - Check the type, strength and expiry date of the local anaesthetic
   - Draw up 10ml using 21G needle
   - Infiltrate the L3/4 or L4/4 vertebral space with a 25G needle
   - Allow a few minutes for the local anaesthetic to work
iii. Insert spinal needle into subarachnoid space
   - Position the spinal needle in the midline between the two spinal processes already identified
   - Advance the needle through the skin with the bevel facing upwards at an angle towards the umbilicus (30 degrees)
   - There will be slight resistance as the needle enters the ligamentum flavum and then a subtle pop when it passes through the dura mater
   - Check that you are in the correct space by removing the stylet of the needle allowing CSF to flow back through the spinal needle
iv. Measure opening pressure
   - Remove the stylet and connect the manometer to the spinal needle and turn the 3 way tap so that the CSF rises up the column
v. Collect CSF into specimen bottles and xanthochromia bottle
   - Turn the tap valve so that CSF in the manometer drains into the specimen bottle 1
   - Collect CSF in sequential specimen bottles (2,3 & 4). Fill the xanthochromia bottle last
vi. Remove the spinal needle and apply a dressing

What would you do at the end of the procedure?

i. Advise the patient to lie on her back for at least 4 hours to reduce the risk of post LP headache
ii. Document the procedure in the notes including the volume of local anaesthetic used

Explain how CSF circulates and is reabsorbed?

- The majority of CSF is produced by the choroid plexus located in the lateral ventricle.
- It circulates from the lateral ventricles into the 3rd ventricle then 4th ventricle before exiting through the foramen of Magendie (medially) and foramen of Luschka (laterally).
- CSF flows in the subarachnoid space around the cerebral hemispheres and spinal cord before being reabsorbed through arachnoid granulation, into dural venous sinuses

Name the layers which the spinal needle passes through to reach the subarachnoid space

i. Skin
ii. Subcutaneous tissue
iii. Supraspinous ligament
iv. Interspinous ligament
v. Ligamentum flavum
vi. Dura mater
vii. Subarachnoid membrane

SURGICAL SKILLS

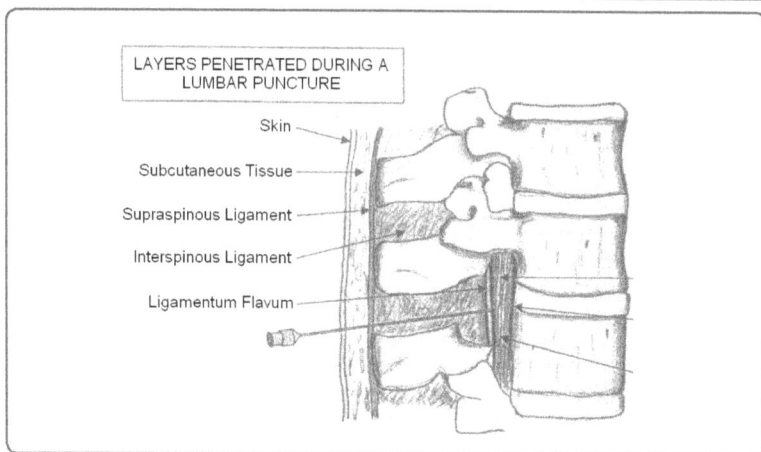

LAYERS PENETRATED DURING A
LUMBAR PUNCTURE

Skin

Subcutaneous Tissue

Supraspinous Ligament

Interspinous Ligament

Ligamentum Flavum

At what spinal level does the spinal cord terminate in adults

- L1/L2

At what spinal level does the subarachnoid space end in adults?

- S2

What is the normal range for opening pressure

- 0-20 cm H2O

What are the contraindications to performing a lumbar puncture

- Relative contraindications
  - Vertebral abnormalities such as scoliosis/kyphosis
  - Presence of infection at puncture site
- Absolute contraindications
  - Patient refusal
  - Severe thrombocytopenia (platelets <50 x 109/L) or coagulopathy
  - Signs and symptoms of raised intra cranial pressure

EXAMINATION SUMMARY

Wash Your Hands
Ensure that you are seen by the examiners to wash your hands using alcohol gel provided.

Introduce, Explain and perform safety checks of patient and consent form
Start by introducing yourself and explaining the procedure. Then perform the essential safety checks of the patient and check the consent form

Prepare equipment and Check local anaesthetic
Check that you have all your equipment available

Position patient and identify the landmarks for insertion
The patient can either be positioned in the sitting or lateral decubitus position. The landmark for insertion is the intervertebral space of L3/L4 or L4/5, which is located at the level of the anterior superior iliac spines

Clean, drape and infiltrate local anaesthetic
Clean the skin, drape using an aseptic technique and infiltrate the local anaesthetic

Insert spinal needle, measure opening pressure and collect CSF
The spinal needle should be inserted into the subarachnoid space by angling toward the umbilicus. Once the correct space is identified collect the manometer and then fill the specimen bottles with CSF

TOP TIPS

➕ There is a lot to complete in this station and in order to finish the procedure you will have to be efficient at performing safety checks and preparing the equipment.

➕ It is not a procedure, which is commonly performed by surgical trainees but can be practised with anaesthetics if they are performing a spinal or epidural in theatre.

➕ The most common questions are around the layers penetrated during a lumbar puncture and possible complications.

SURGICAL SKILLS

2.14 | Male Urethral Catheterisation

> ## Scenario
>
> A 60 year old man presents to A&E with acute urinary retention. You are the on-call urology trainee and the A&E triage nurse has asked you to insert a urethral catheter. Please perform this procedure

Describe what you do before starting the procedure

Start by introducing yourself and checking the patient, consent form and explaining the procedure

i. Introduce yourself
ii. Patient checks
- Confirm the patients' name and date of birth
- Check if there have been any previous catheterisation attempts, urinary tract instrumentation or prostate surgery
- Check if they are on any medications and their allergy status (especially to latex)
    - If the patient has latex allergy ensure that a 100% silicone catheter is used and non-latex gloves
- Request a bladder scan
iii. Obtain consent
- Explain that you will start by cleaning the penis then insert some gel as a local anaesthetic. You will then pass a thin flexible tube into the bladder.
- The benefit is that this will allow him to pass urine
- The risks are discomfort both during and after the procedure due to bladder spasms, risk of infection, bleeding, false passage and failed procedure
iv. Offer a chaperone
- Normally you would want a nurse to be present to both help and chaperone

What equipment will you need for the procedure?

The following equipment will be needed
i. Sterile gloves
ii. Catheter pack containing a kidney disk, gauze, gallipot and sterile drape
iii. Skin preparation solution (saline or sterile water)
iv. Instillagel 10ml
v. Appropriate Foley catheter (14Fr or 16Fr)
vi. 10ml syringe with water (may be supplied with catheter
vii. Catheter bag

How would you position the patient for the procedure

The patient should be lying as flat as possible with legs flat. He should be exposed from xipherstum to below the knee but keep the patient covered with a sheet until starting the procedure to maintain dignity.

Demonstrate how you would perform the procedure

i. Clean and drape
- Wash hands and put on sterile gloves
- Use non-dominant hand to retract foreskin
- Clean the glans and meatus with gauze soaked in skin preparation solution
- Apply sterile drape
ii. Instillagel

- Hold penis proximal to the corona between index finger and thumb with non-dominant hand
- Stretch the penis upwards towards the ceiling
- Instil 10ml instillagel after warning the patient that it may feel cold and sting a bit
- Say that you would wait 3-5 mins for instillagel with the penis held upright

iii. Insert catheter
- Hold penis upright with non-dominant hand
- Pass the catheter with gentle traction into the urethra using your dominant hand
- Continue passing the catheter until you feel gentle resistance at the bulbar urethra
- At this point the penis can be lowered
- Continuing inserting catheter until the hilt is at the meatus and allow urine to drain
- Only after urine has started draining should you inflate the balloon with 10ml water and retract catheter
- Connect the catheter bag
- Replace the foreskin

What would you do at the end of the procedure?

i. Document the procedure in the notes including
- Type and size of catheter with sticker if aviallable
- Description of urine (colour, present of sediment)
- Residual volume

ii. Take a urine sample for MC&S

If no urine drains after inserting the catheter what would you?

- The key thing to say is that you would not inflate the balloon unless urine has started to drain.
- If no urine is draining you can apply gentle suprapubic pressure and aspirate with a syringe
- If these manoeuvres fail the catheter can be washed out using a bladder syringe and a small volume (50ml) sterile water

What is the average length of the male urethra?

- 20cm (8 inches) long

Name the parts of the male urethra

- Posterior urethra which includes prostatic urethra and membranous urethra
- Anterior urethra which includes bulbar urethra, penile urethra, fossa navicularis and urethral meatus

Where is the narrowest part of the urethra?

- The external orifice at the glans penis is the narrowest part of the male urethra

What does a 18Fr catheter size refer to

- The French (Fr) size is a measure of the diameter of the catheter
- One French is equivalent to 0.33mm so the diameter of the catheter can be calculated by dividing the French size by 3. An 18Fr catheter has a diameter of 6mm.

SURGICAL SKILLS

What can be done if a catheter cannot be passed easily through the prostatic urethra

- A Coudé tip catheter a bend at the distal end which can be used to negotiate a high bladder neck secondary to benign prostatic hypertrophy
- If this does not easily pass the catheter should be inserted under direct vision with flexible cystoscopy
- If all these manoeuvres fail then a suprapubic catheter can be inserted

What other types of catheters do you know

- Robinson (straight) catheter – these are designed as once only 'in and out' catheters
- Foley catheter – the most common catheter characterised a self-retaining balloon at the distal end
- Three-way catheter – these are triple catheters containing and inflow and outflow port as well as a port for balloon inflation

SUMMARY

Wash Your Hands
Ensure that you are seen by the examiners to wash your hands using alcohol gel provided.

Introduce, Explain and perform safety checks of patient and consent form
Start by introducing yourself and explaining the procedure. Then perform the essential patient checks, explain the procedure and take consent

Prepare equipment
Check that you have all your equipment available

Position and expose the patient
The patient should be supine and exposed from xiphsternum to below the knees. Ensure he is covered until the procedure begins to maintain dignity

Clean, drape and infiltrate instillagel
Retract the foreskin, clean the glans, drape using an aseptic technique and infiltrate 10ml instillagel

Insert catheter
The catheter should be inserted with the penis held upright until it reaches the bulbar urethra. Insert the catheter to the hilt and only inflate the balloon once urine has started to drain

SURGICAL SKILLS

TOP TIPS

✚ This is a relatively simple procedure to perform and you should be prepared for more questions at the end of the station

✚ It is important to be aware of sterile technique and keeping one hand 'clean'. Alternatively a double glove technique can be used

✚ The procedure will be performed on a model which often feel very different to normal catheterisation. Try to practice with a model as you may find that more force is required to pass the catheter due to lack of lubrication.

SURGICAL SKILLS

2.15 | Needle Thoracostomy

Scenario

You attend a trauma call for a 44 year old woman who has been involved in a road traffic accident. You are asked to insert a traumatic chest drain.

You are shown her chest x-ray. What is the diagnosis?

This is an AP erect chest x-ray
- There are absent left lung markings and the mediastinum is shifted to the right
- There is no evidence of rib fractures
- This is consistent with a left sided tension pneumothorax – this should have been detected clinically prior to a chest x-ray

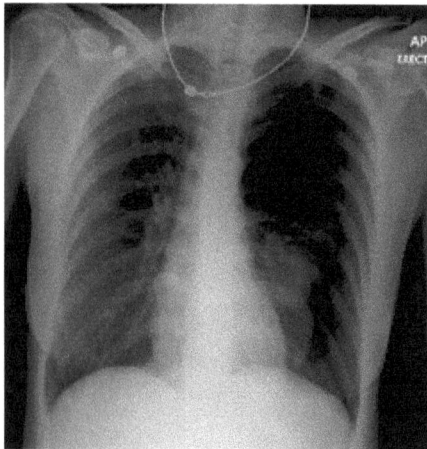

What signs and symptoms may be clinically apparent

- Tracheal deviation to the right
- Distended neck veins
- Severe SOB, tachycardia & hypotension

What procedure is required?

Emergency needle thoracostomy followed by insertion of traumatic chest drain

Describe how you would perform a needle thoracostomy

- A 16G cannula is inserted into the second intercostal space of the left side in the mid-clavicular line
- The cannula is inserted 90 degrees to skin into the pleural space
- The needle is withdrawn with a characteristic rush of air.
- The cannula is left open and secured in the chest

Describe what you do before starting the chest drain insertion

i. Introduce yourself
ii. Patient checks
   * Confirm the patients' name and date of birth
   * Check if they are on any medications, especially anticoagulants, and their allergy status
   * Prophylactic antibiotics: BTS guidelines recommend prophylactic antibiotics for all traumatic chest drains
iii. Consent form
   * Check the consent form and that it is signed and dated
   * If the patient is not able to consent then a consent form 4 should be completed and signed by the most senior medical professional present

What equipment will you need for the procedure?

The following equipment will be needed
i.   Sterile gloves and gown
ii.   Skin preparation solution (e.g. chlorheixidne),
iii. Local anaesthetic (1% lignocaine) and 10ml syringe
iv.   21G (Green) needle and 25G (orange) needle
v.   No. 11 blade with handle
vi.   Spencer wells clamp or large forceps for blunt dissection
vii. Drain clamp
viii. Large bore chest drain (<24Hr)
ix.   Suture material (Silk 1-0)
x.   Connecting tubing
xi.   Closed drainage system
xii. Occlusive dressing

How would *you* position the patient and identify the landmarks for insertion

i. Position: At 45 degrees with right arm above head (to expose insertion site)
ii. Insertion site at 5th intercostal space just anterior to midaxillary line within the safe triangle of insertion

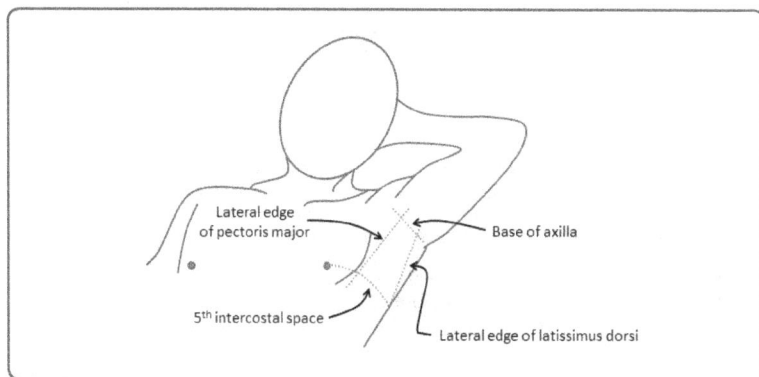

Lateral edge of pectoris major

Base of axilla

5th intercostal space

Lateral edge of latissimus dorsi

Demonstrate how you would perform the procedure

i. Clean and drape
   * Prepare the skin with chlorhexidine 2%
   * Drape the patient using an aseptic technique
ii. Local anaesthetic

SURGICAL SKILLS

- Check the type, strength and expiry date of the local anaesthetic
- Draw up 10ml using 21G needle
- Infiltrate the insertion site with 25G needle
- Allow a few minutes for the local anaesthetic to work

iii. Incision and dissection to pleura
- Make 2-3cm transverse incision just above 6th rib to avoid damage to intercostal bundles
- Blunt dissection through the tissues using Spencer wells clamp or large forceps
- Puncture the parietal pleura using Spencer wells clamp
- Perform a finger sweep to ensure there are no adhesions

iv. Insertion of chest drain
- Clamp drain and place below patient
- Pass tube aiming apically for a pneumothorax
- Observe the tube for fogging to confirm appropriate placement
- Connect to underwater seal drainage system
- Check fluid in tube is moving with respiration (swinging) and bubbling

v. Secure chest drain
- Using 1-0 silk perform two sutures
  - A horizontal mattress suture to close the wound after drain removal
  - A stay suture to secure the drain.
- Apply the occlusive dressing

What would you do at the end of the procedure?

i. Request a chest x-ray to confirm the correct placement of the chest drain
ii. Document the procedure in the notes including volume of local anaesthetic, the chest drain size, the type of suture and knot used.
iii. The patient should have regular observations and particularly pulse oximetry. The chest drain should be monitored for continued swinging and bubbling

What are the complications of inserting a chest drain

- Early complication
  - Damage to intercostal nerves (can cause intercostal neuralgia) or long thoracic nerve
  - Damage to intercostal veins & arteries (can convert pneumothorax to haemthorax)
  - Damage to organs (e.g. liver), heart or lungs
  - Malposition:
- Late complications
  - Blocked tube
  - Empyema
  - Pneumothorax following removal

What is the boundaries of the safe triangle

i. Posterior margin: Mid-axillary line to avoid long thoracic nerve
ii. Anterior Margin: Lateral border of Pectoralis Major
iii. Inferior Margin: 5th intercostal space
iv. Apex: Below axilla

What do you look for to confirm that the chest drain is functioning

- Swinging: The fluid level in the drain will rise and fall with respiration
- Bubbling in the underwater seal

What would you do if the drain stopes swinging

- Check the dressing and exit site to ensure it is not kinked
- Inspect the tubing for blockage with clots of thick secretions.
- Perform a chest x-ray to check if the drain is appropriately placed

When would you remove this chest drain

- When the chest drain has stopped bubbling and the chest ray confirms lung re-expansion

What respiratory manoeuvre should the patient perform as the chest drain is being removed

- The BTS guidelines say that chest drains should be removed either during expiration or with the Valsalva manoeuvre

EXAMINATION SUMMARY

Wash Your Hands
Ensure that you are seen by the examiners to wash your hands using alcohol gel provided.

Perform needle thoracostomy
Insert a 16G cannula into the second intercostal space in the midclavicular line

Pre-procedure checks
Check patient's identification, give prophylactic antibiotics and check the consent form

Prepare equipment for chest drain insertion
Check that you have all your equipment available

Position patient and identify the landmarks for insertion
The patient should be at 45 degrees with their ipsilateral arm above their head
The insertion site is the 5th intercostal space just anterior to the mid-axiallary line

Clean, drape and infiltrate local anaesthetic
Clean the skin, drape using an aseptic technique and infiltrate the local anaesthetic

Insert chest drain
Make incision above 6th rib and dissect down to the parietal pleura. Puncture the pleura and perform a finger sweep. Pass the chest drain towards the apex and check for fogging. Connect the underwater seal

Secure chest drain
Perform a horizontal mattress suture and stay suture with 1-0 Silk. Apply an occlusive dressing

SURGICAL SKILLS

TOP TIPS

+ The main challenge with this station is completing the procedure in the timeframe

+ You can save time by quickly interpreting the chest x-ray and preparing your equipment. Ask the examiner to help as an assistance in case you forget anything

+ The procedure will be performed on a model and it is good to practice with the model as the tissues feel different. Generally they require more force for blunt dissection that would be advised in a human

+ Make sure you learn the boundaries of the safe triangle and insertion site well.

SURGICAL SKILLS

2.16 | Organising a List A

Scenario

You are the surgical registrar and your consultant has asked you to organise the following patients on the theatre list. Please inform the theatre co-ordinator of the order.

Name	Hospital Number	Sex	Age	Operation	Comments
AM	745931	F	68	Laparoscopic right hemicolectomy	Allergy to penicillin and iodine
IW	472007	M	63	Hartmanns procedure for perforated diverticular abscess	Left THR
JD	599814	M	72	Open right inguinal hernia repair	Severe COPD
JS	204956	M	54	Laparoscopic cholecystectomy	Pacemaker and on warfarin

Please state your order and the reasons behind your choice?

I would place the patients in the following order:
1) IW (perforated diverticular abscess)
I would place this patient first as they are likely to be unwell due to their diverticular abscess and require urgent surgery.
2) AM (laparoscopic hemicolectomy)
As this is the next major procedure it should ideally be done earlier in the day.
3) JD (open inguinal hernia repair)
This patient suffers from severe COPD and would need to be prioritised.
4) JS (laparoscopic cholecystectomy)
I would place this patient last as they are undergoing a less major procedure with no severe co-morbidities. Placing the patient last will give the team time, if necessary, to ensure the inr is checked and within range and allow any pacemaker checks that need to be done

SURGICAL SKILLS

How would you classify surgical emergencies?

Surgical emergencies can be classified according to the National Confidential Enquiry into Patient Outcome and Death (NECPOD) Classification of Intervention, as summarised in the following table.

Code	Category	Description	Target time to theatre	Examples
1	Immediate	– Life, limb or organ saving surgery – Simultaneous resuscitation and surgical treatment	– Within minutes of decisi67on to operate – Next available theatre or break into existing theatre list	– Ruptured abdominal aortic aneurysm – Compartment syndrome – Major thoraco-abdominal trauma – Fracture with neurovascular deficit – Acute myocardial infarction
2	Urgent	– Acute onset or deterioration of conditions that threaten life, limbs or organ survival – Injuries requiring fracture fixation – Surgical treatment usually preformed when resuscitation is complete	– Within hours of decision to operate – Emergency lists (daytime or out-of-hours)	– Open fracture – Critical organ or limb ischaemia – Perforated bowel with peritonitis – Acute coronary syndrome
3	Expedited	– Stable patient requiring early intervention for a condition which is not an immediate threat to life, limb or organ survival – Emergency day lists or elective lists with spare capacity	– Within days of decision to operate	– Tendon and nerve injuries
4	Elective	– Procedures for conditions requiring routine hospital admission	– Booked or planned in advance – Elective theatre lists	– All procedure not classified as in the above categories

What is the ASA grading system?

This is a system devised by the American Society of Anesthesiologists (ASA) that categorises patients into groups according to their co-morbid burden.

ASA Grade	Definition	Examples
I	Normal healthy individual	– Non-smoking – Minimal alcohol intake
II	Mild systemic disease with no functional limitation	– Smoker – Social alcohol intake – Pregnancy – Obesity – Well controlled diabetes/hypertension – Mild lung disease
III	Severe systemic disease with functional limitation	– Alcohol dependence – Morbidly obese – Poorly controlled diabetes/hypertension – COPD – Moderate reduction of ejection fraction – History of MI, CVA, TIA, cardiac stents (>3 months) – End stage renal disease undergoing regular dialysis
IV	Severe systemic disease which is a constant threat to life	– Severe reduction of ejection fraction – History of MI, CVA, TIA, cardiac stents (<3 months) – End stage renal disease not undergoing regular dialysis – Ongoing cardiac ischaemia or severe valve dysfunction – Sepsis – DIC
V	Moribund and not expected to survive 24 hours	– Ruptured AAA – Massive trauma – Intracranial bleed with mass effect – Ischaemic bowel with significant cardiac disease or multiple organ disease

Describe the various abdominal incisions and associated procedures.

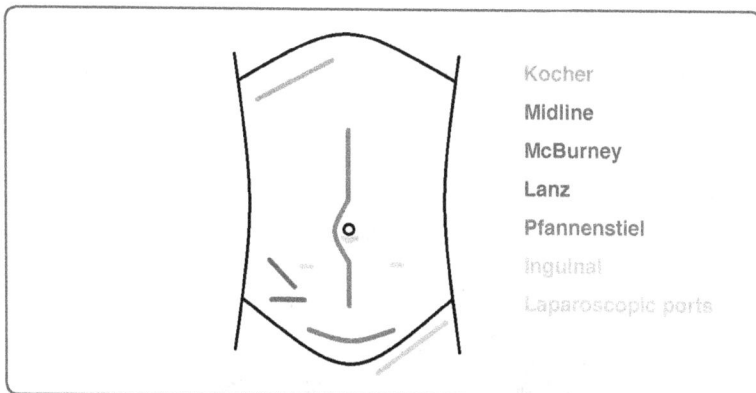

Kocher

Midline

McBurney

Lanz

Pfannenstiel

Inguinal

Laparoscopic ports

SURGICAL SKILLS

What are the indications for a Hartmann's procedure?

A Hartmann's procedure is where the rectosigmoid colon is resected with closure of the rectal stump and formation of an end-colostomy. Indications include:
– Obstruction
– Bowel perforation
– Rectosigmoid carcinoma
– Trauma

What considerations would you have to make when placing a stoma?

– Avoid bony prominences, skin creases, belt lines and scars
– It should be placed in an area that is easy for the patient to manage
– It should be placed through the rectus femoris to reduce the likelihood of herniation

What pre-operative considerations would you make in patient JD?

Pre-operative investigations – blood tests, ECG and a CXR. Lung function tests and ABGs. Pre-operative interventions – smoking cessation, physiotherapy to improve lung function, corticosteroids and antibiotics to treat acute exacerbations and nebulisers to reduce bronchospasm.

What considerations would be made intra-operatively for patient JD?

In severe COPD a spinal anaesthetic may be administered. In milder cases of COPD it is possible to give a general anaesthetic supplemented with intermittent positive pressure ventilation.

Are there any post-operative considerations for patient JD?

Yes. There are various levels of post-operative care (see table below) and patient JD may require an HDU bed due to their severe COPD possibly needing ventilator support. Patients will require adequate analgesia to allow deep breathing to prevent chest infections, in addition to chest physiotherapy to clear secretions and being nursed upright.

Level	Setting	Description	Nurse:patient ratio
0	Normal ward	Unmonitored beds	Variable
1	Enhanced care	Monitored bed	3:1
2	HDU	Single organ failure No ventilation requirement	2:1
3	ITU	Multi-organ failure Ventilated	1:1

When are prophylactic antibiotics indicated?

Prophylactic antibiotics prevent bacteria from multiplying without affecting the normal tissue flora and have a role in preventing surgical site infections. They are usually administered as a single dose within 30 minutes of anaesthesia to allow adequate time for levels to accumulate in tissue, as high levels of antibiotics need to be obtained at the time of the procedure. They are indicated in:

– Patients who are immunocompromised or have prosthetic heart valves to prevent

endocarditis
- Procedures where prophylactic antibiotics have proven evidence in reducing post-operative infections e.g. insertion of implants or in procedures that commonly lead to infection such as colectomies

What skin preparations would you use in the above patients?

Patient AM is allergic to iodine and therefore chlorhexadine should be used. Either iodine or chlorhexadine could be used in the others patients.

What is diathermy and explain the different types?

Diathermy is the use of high-frequency electrical currents to produce heat to cut tissue or coagulate vessels. There are different modes including:
Cutting: low frequency currents through a continuous out-put
Coagulation: high frequency currents through a pulsed out-put
Blend: continuous current with bursts of high intensity current

Monopolar diathermy is where the electrical current passes from the instrument (active electrode with high current density) through the patient back to the generator (low current density) via an electrode placed on the patient. It is a high power unit (400W) that generates high frequencies. Bipolar diathermy uses a current that passes between two electrodes, usually between the tips of forceps where a patient electrode is not needed. It is a low power unit (50W) generating low frequencies.

Complications of diathermy can include burns particularly when used with alcohol based preparations, electrocution and interference with pacemaker function. Bipolar diathermy is safer and is useful on surgery to the extremities but has no cutting or buzzing capability.

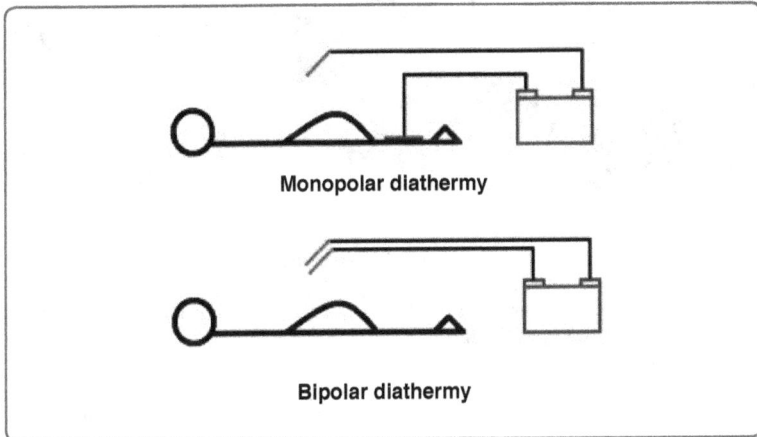

Monopolar diathermy

Bipolar diathermy

What considerations have to be made when placing diathermy pads?

Diathermy pads must be placed away from bony prominences and scars as they can cause burns. It is also important to place away from other metalwork e.g. prostheses. They should be placed on dry, shaved skin with at least 70cm² contact surface area.

What would you have to consider in a patient with a pacemaker?

The various theatre team members should be aware of a patient with a pacemaker.

Diathermy can interfere with the pacing function so it is important to use bipolar diathermy The diathermy pad should be placed away from the pacemaker so current flowing between the diathermy and patient electrode is not near the pacemaker. The anaesthetist must also ensure adequate monitoring and availability of equipment if there is a functional failure of the pacing device.

What are the indications for drains in surgery?

Drains are indicated in established or anticipated collections. They are also used to minimise dead space and prevent fluid from collecting e.g. following a mastectomy or when there is risk of a leak e.g. bowel anastomoses. They can also be used to decompress compartments e.g. pneumothorax. Drains can either be open or closed systems, the latter which reduces the risk of introducing infection, or they can be or suction or non-suction drains, where suction drains can damage adjacent structures but do provide better drainage.

SUMMARY

As a general rule patients placed first on lists are usually children, diabetics and clean surgeries. Traditionally those placed last are infected cases or patients with MRSA to allow sufficient time for theatre cleaning. Patients undergoing major surgery or those with complex anaesthetic issues or significant co-morbidities tend to be earlier. However, clinical urgency is priority regardless of these factors.

TOP TIPS

➕ It is not necessarily the correct order that scores marks, but the reason behind your decision and appreciating urgency of procedure, co-morbidities, presence of infection etc that the examiner will look for.

References:
The NCEPOD Classification of Intervention. 2004. Available URL: http://www.ncepod.org.uk/pdf/NCEPODClassification.pdf
American Society of Anaesthesiologists. 2014 ASA Physical Status Classification System. Available URL: https://www.asahq.org/resources/clinical-information/asa-physical-status-classification-system
McCloy R, Thomas B, Weston J. 2012. Electrosurgery. *Intercollegiate Basic Surgical Skills Course Participant Handbook.* London. The Royal College of Surgeons of England, pp. 45-57.

2.17 | Organising a List B

Scenario

You are the night orthopaedic registrar oncall and have to submit the trauma list to the theatre coordinator. Please order the following patients.

Name	Hospital Number	Sex	Age	Operation	Comments
JP	660324	F	81	Left hip hemiarthroplasty	PPM, HTN, angina, previous CVA
VK	601729	M	64	Left DHS	Warfarin for a metallic valve
TJ	409846	M	33	Right open tibia fracture	Latex allergy
WW	710902	M	70	Right BKA	IDDM and MRSA

State the order of patients and justify your order.

1) TJ (open tibia fracture).
This patient has an open fracture that requires urgent surgical intervention, they also have a latex allergy and ideally should be placed first on the list.
2) JP (hip hemiarthroplasty).
This patient is older and due to their co-morbidities I would place them next on the list.
3) VK (DHS).
I would place this patient next as the last case is a dirty case and consideration needs to be made to the use of implants.
WW (BKA).
This patient has MRSA and should be placed last on the list unless there was a life or limb threatening concern. Although they have IDDM and should be placed earlier on the list given the information the other patients should be prioritised.

How would you position each of the above patients?

JP: Right lateral position
VK: Traction table
TJ: Supine
WW: Supine

Correct positioning should allow adequate exposure of the surgical field and minimise injuries to patients. It should also facilitate anaesthetic administration and monitoring to maintain breathing, circulation and physiological requirement.

SURGICAL SKILLS

Position	Patient placement	Example
Supine	Back	Majority of surgeries – Abdominal – Upper and lower limb (with the use of arm board, sand bags, supports etc)
Prone	Front	– Spinal – Intracranial – Achilles tendon repair
Lateral	Side	– Hip – Thoracic
Trendelenburg	Supine with head down	– Lower abdominal (allows intestines to move away from the pelvis due to gravity) – Gynaecological – Urological – Colorectal – Pelvic
Reverse trendelenburg	Supine with head up	– Upper abdominal – Head and neck
Lithotomy	Supine with hips and knees flexed and ankles supported in stirrups	– Gynaecological – Urological – Colorectal – Pelvic
Lloyd Davies	Similar to lithotomy but calves supported in pneumatic stirrups	As above
Beech-chair		– Shoulder – Intracranial (posterior fossa)

What injuries can arise from positioning of patients?

All members of the operating team should be aware of the common injuries that can arise secondary to the positioning of patients and therefore put measures in place to avoid this. Nerve injuries can result from compression, stretching and ischaemia. Commonly injured nerves include ulnar (compression of the medial epicondyle and the edge of the table in a pronated arm), radial (compression of the humeral shaft against the edge of the table) and common peroneal (compression of the fibula neck and the edge of the operating table particularly in the lithotomy or Lloyd Davies position). Superficial skin injuries can arise from sticky drapes and electrodes to more severe insult from diathermy burns, pressure sores and allergic reactions to skin preparations. Injuries can also occur from those related to anaesthesia including damage to teeth during intubation and corneal abrasions that can be prevented by taping the eyelids closed.

How are theatres designed and how does the filtration of theatre air differ for these patients?

Operating theatres should be located adjacent to ITU and close to surgical wards with minimal distance to the Emergency Department and radiology. There are four areas within an operating suite an outer general access zone (reception and general offices), a clean limited access area (area between reception and theatres), a restricted access zone (for those that are appropriately dressed, the anaesthetic area and scrub rooms) and the aseptic zone which is the theatre itself.

Air within theatre is filtered from air outside of theatre to remove microscopic particles. To maintain minimum microorganism counts there should be a minimum number of air changes per hour.

There are two types of airflow:

Turbulent and laminar – In turbulent flow theatres a positive pressure current with random airflow is generated in the operating room causing a decreased pressure compared to the exterior. This ensures airborne organisms are carried out.

Laminar – There is positive pressure with parallel airflow, where peripheral theatre vents filter air that is pumped into theatre preventing contaminated air from re-entering. Additional fans producing downwards airflow under the laminar flow hood helps remove contamination generated around the wound and exposed instruments. It also prevents air from the theatre periphery entering to under the canopy, usually with more air changes per hour. In general, trauma and orthopaedic surgery particularly with the use of implants and metalwork is preformed in laminar flow theatres which are thought to reduce the rate of surgical site infections.

What consideration would you have to make if patient JP had dementia.

Assess capacity to see if they were able to consent to a procedure. The Mental Capacity Act 2005 states a person lacks capacity if they are unable to make a specific decision, at a specific time because of an impairment or disturbance in the functioning of the brain or mind.

Capacity can change in patients and it is important to check capacity regularly. To be able to make a decision a person should be able to:

– Understand the decision to be made and information provided regarding the decision.
– Retain the information provided long enough to make the decision.
– Use the information provided to make a decision by weighing up pros and cons.
– Communicate their decision.

Check if patients have an advanced directive

What are the various consent forms?

Consent Form	Use
1	Patient agreement to investigation, treatment or procedure
2	Parental agreement to investigation, treatment or procedure for a child or young person
3	Patient/parental agreement to investigation, treatment or procedure (where consciousness is not impaired)
4	Form for adults who are unable to consent to investigation or treatment

The legal age of consent is 16 and those below this age require a parent or a legal guardian to provide consent on their behalf.

In the case of refusal, the decision can be overridden by a doctor if acting in their best interests where a court order must be obtained. Children under 16 can provide consent if they are deemed competent (Gillick competent) but cannot refuse a procedure where a parent or legal guardian can authorise treatment. In cases where expressed consent cannot be gained if the patient is unconscious for example, surgery can still be preformed if it is thought to be in the best interests of the patient.

What do you have to consider in patient VK?

This patient is on warfarin for a mechanical valve. Reversing the effect of warfarin prior to surgery needs to be carefully considered in the presence of a mechanical valve by following local guidelines or discussing with the haematology team.

How do you manage patients on warfarin prior to surgery?

Warfarin management differs in the elective and emergency patient and surgery is usually safely preformed when the INR is less than 2. In elective surgery warfarin is usually stopped 4-5 days prior to surgery, with LMWH injections to act as bridging therapy. However, in those patients where anticoagulation is critical an intravenous heparin infusion should be commenced, regularly monitoring the APTT to ensure it is in therapeutic range. The heparin should be stopped prior to surgery and recommenced immediately after. Warfarin is restarted when the patient is eating and the heparin is stopped once the INR is in range. In emergency surgery vitamin K is given.

How would you classify open fractures?

The Gustilo and Anderson classification describes open fractures based on associated soft tissue injury.

Gustilo Anderson Grade	Wound size	Soft tissue injury	Energy level
I	<1cm	Minimal	Low
II	1-10cm	Moderate	Moderate
IIIa	>10cm	Extensive with adequate cover	High
IIIb		Extensive with inadequate cover	
IIIc		Extensive with arterial injury	

How would you debride a wound?

The degree of micro and macro-contamination should be considered when debriding wounds. Wounds should be thoroughly washed. Use increasing litres of saline wash with increasing degrees of contamination. When removing devitalised tissue it is important to assess the viability of:
– Skin through capillary refill time, bleeding from the dermis and colour
– Muscle through colour, capillary bleeding and contractility by sqeezing the muscle with forceps
– Bone via the degree of periosteal stripping and bleeding from debrided edges

What would you be concerned about patient TJ developing?

I would be concerned about the development of compartment syndrome. Compartment syndrome is when there is increased interstitial pressure within a closed myofascial compartment resulting in microvascular compromise. The most important symptom is pain out of proportion to the injury and the most important sign is pain on passive stretch of the compartment. Other more late signs and symptoms include paralysis, paraesthesia, pallor and absent peripheral pulses. It is a clinical diagnosis and if there is a strong suspicion fasciotomies should be preformed to decompress the compartment. It is possible to measure intracompartmental pressures (ICP) with fasciotomy indicated when the absolute ICP>30mmHg or there is a difference of <30mmHg between diasytolic blood pressure and ICP.

What is the difference between a graft and a flap and what is the reconstructive ladder?

A graft and flap is a unit of tissue which is moved from a donor to recipient site.

Flap has an attached arterial and venous supply.

Graft is dependent on a good vascular bed for survival.

The reconstructive ladder is the approach to restoring normal structure and function of tissues:

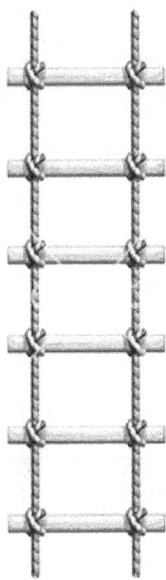

Free flap
A flap which is transferred and anastomosed from one body area to another.
Example: latissimus dorsi or transverse rectus abdominis musculocutaneous flap for breast reconstruction.

Local flap
Rotational: a flap moved sideways to fill a triangular defect which already exists or is created to ensure there is no secondary defect.
Advancement: a flap which is formed and stretched to fill a defect.
Transposition: similar to a rotation flap but where a secondary defect is formed using a split thickness graft.
Example: coverage of an amputation.

Grafts
Split thickness: epidermis and variable amount of dermis, where donor sites have the ability to reepithelialise so do not require closure.
Example: burns.
Full thickness: epidermis and entire dermis with no regenerative capability so donor sites require closure
Example: facial defects that require tissue for contouring

Primary intention
Direct primary closure: healing occurs by connective tissue deposition and epithelialisation through the use of sutures or staples for closure.
Example: lacerations.
Delayed primary closure: wound closure several days after injury due to contamination.
Example: contaminated open fractures with adequate soft tissue cover not requiring a graft or flap.

Secondary intention
The wound is left open to heal by granulation tissue formation, contraction of wound edges and epithelialisation, this may be assisted by dressings. In simple superficial wounds, wound edges maybe approximated by the use of steristrips.
Example: venous leg ulcers.

SURGICAL SKILLS

What considerations have to made in patients with latex allergies?

Patients should ideally be placed first on the list, however if there are other patients requiring more urgent surgery then sufficient time should be allowed for latex particles to settle and the theatre should be thoroughly cleaned. Theatre staff should be informed so latex-containing items are removed from theatre and the sterile surgical services department should also be informed so latex-containing items are not mixed with non-latex items. All staff in contact with the patient should use latex free gloves.

Describe the use of tourniquets.

Tourniquets are commonly used in orthopaedic surgery to provide a bloodless operative field. This is achieved by applying an occlusive band proximal to the operative site that reduces blood flow to the limb. It is important to use appropriate sized cuffs for the limb and patient and adequately pad beneath it. Specialised rubber band tourniquets are available for digital surgery. Tourniquets are usually inflated to 100-150mmHg above the systolic blood pressure. 50mmHg above systolic in the arm and 100mmHg above systolic in the lower limb. The maximum time a tourniquet must be applied to the upper limb is 60-90mins and the lower limb 90-120mins. Prolonged use may be obtained by a period of deflation (for 10mins) and re-inflation to allow reperfusion. Contraindications to their use include peripheral vascular disease, vasculitic disorders, previous thrombo-embolic events, previous vascular surgery on the limb to be operated on and sickle cell disease.

What are the indications for an amputation and what factors do you have to consider for the level of amputation?

An amputation of a limb is indicated if it is non-viable, this may result from arterial or venous disease, diabetes, infection or trauma.

The level of amputation depends on the viability of: 1) soft tissue and its coverage, 2) bone and 3) its vascular supply which can clinically be assessed by temperature, colour and atrophic changes or measured through Doppler scans. Other factors that must be considered for the level of amputation include underlying pathology, cosmetic appearance and the patient's functional requirement and ability to rehabilitate.

SUMMARY

Whilst there are general rules to organising theatre lists with regards to patient factors as discussed in Organising a List A, surgeons must be aware of various other factors that affect planning of surgery including having the relevant equipment/implants available, need for image guidance etc.

TOP TIPS

✚ Try to practice ordering lists by asking seniors to test your knowledge.

References:
Department of Health. 2009. Consent forms. Available URL http://webarchive.nationalarchives.gov.uk/+/www.dh.gov.uk/en/publichealth/scientificdevelopmentgeneticsandbioethics/consent/consentgeneralinformation/DH_4015950

SURGICAL SKILLS

2.18 | Removal of a Naevus

Scenario

You are the surgical registrar and you are with your consultant in day case theatre. The next patient is a 25 year old lady attending for removal of a naevus on her arm. The patient is prepped and draped and local anaesthetic has been administered. Your consultant has been called away for an emergency and you have been asked to continue. You will find a nurse assistant on entering the station.

How will you proceed?

– Wash hands, introduce yourself and explain the procedure
– Re-do WHO surgical checklist
– Check site, consent form and wristband
– Check allergies
– Ensure correct patient positioning, prep and draping
– Check skin anaesthetised
– Mark elliptical incision length 3-4 times compared with width (to gain adequate margins)
– Excise lesion, close and dress wound
– Dispose of sharps safely
– Send specimen for histology, label forms and pot
– Explain post-operative care
– Complete operation note

What local anaesthetic and dose would you use?

Lignocaine or lignocaine with adrenaline could be used as the lesion is on the arm and not near end arteries. The maximum safe dose of lignocaine is 3mg/kg and 6mg/kg of lignocaine with adrenaline. When administering anaesthetic there are two techniques. The 'static' method is where the needle is inserted in the area requiring anaesthetising and then aspirated to ensure no blood is drawn back from entrance into a vessel which could cause cardiac dysrhythmias if intravenously injected. Alternatively the needle maybe continuously moved through the tissue so any penetration into a blood vessel would be transient and a significant volume intravenous injection would be avoided. It is best practice to start with a fine bore needle and then change to a longer, large-bore needle for deeper infiltration ensuring the initial planned area of surgery is anaesthetised.

What is the effect of adrenaline in local anaesthetic?

Adrenaline acts to slow systemic absorption by overcoming vasodilatory action, therefore prolonging the duration of activity so higher doses can be used. It also reduces bleeding but should not be used in end arteries.

Why is it important to check the anaesthetic is working?

Local anaesthetic blocks transmission of action potentials in nerve cells by reversibly blocking Na channels. Unmyelinated C fibres (smaller nerve fibres) are more sensitive and may need higher doses to block pain transmission. This is sometimes why patients feel pressure but not pain and is known as differential conduction blockade and explains why nerve blocks should be tested prior to surgery.

SURGICAL SKILLS

Explain how you would excise the lesion?

– Mark an elliptical incision over the lesion, which measured to allow adequate margins and enough clearance on each side. The long axis of the lesion is multiplied by three to get the length of the incision, which is the minimum calculated width to length ratio for a cosmetic closure without tension.
– Excise the marked area with the blade perpendicular to the skin including the lesion with a portion of subcutaneous tissue.
– Close the wound with interrupted vertical mattress sutures starting at alternate ends and advancing to the centre of the excised area.

Describe your dissection technique.

There are two types of dissection technique. Sharp dissection uses tissue scissors or a knife to undermine skin and toothed forceps help elevate the skin. Blunt dissection is where the tissue is carefully separated by the fingers, swabs or blunt instruments.

How could you aid closure of an elliptical wound?

It is possible to undermine wound edges to help closure. Placing skin hooks can help to display the wound. Ensuring the length of the wound is approximately three times the width of the wound will minimise the amount of tension placed on the wound.

How would you close the wound?

I would close the wound with interrupted non absorbable sutures.

What post-operative instructions would you give?

– When the wound should be checked and sutures removed
– Clinic appointment
– How long to keep the dressings on e.g. 48 hours
– How to keep it clean
– What factors to look for the development of infection

What are the common blade types you will encounter?

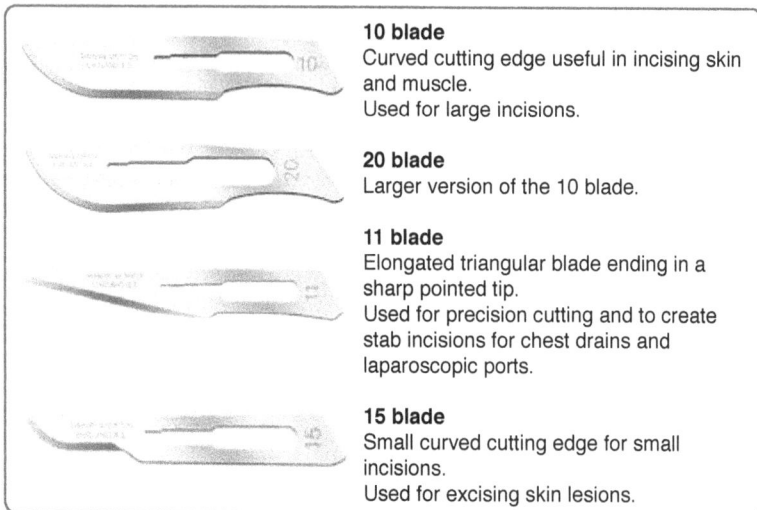

10 blade
Curved cutting edge useful in incising skin and muscle.
Used for large incisions.

20 blade
Larger version of the 10 blade.

11 blade
Elongated triangular blade ending in a sharp pointed tip.
Used for precision cutting and to create stab incisions for chest drains and laparoscopic ports.

15 blade
Small curved cutting edge for small incisions.
Used for excising skin lesions.

SURGICAL SKILLS

Can you describe a prognostic factor in skin melanoma?

The most important prognostic factor in malignant melanoma is tumour thickness. Breslow's thickness measures how deeply tumours have invaded from the granular layer of the epidermis to the deepest point of tumour infiltration in the vertical plane.

Depth (mm)	5-year survival (%)
<1	9-99
1.01-2.0	8-90
2.01-4	6-75
>4	<50

What is the WHO checklist?

The WHO checklist is a checklist designed to minimise the most common and avoidable risks in surgery that could cause harm to the patient. It is composed of three steps to decrease errors and adverse events. The WHO checklist has been shown to significantly reduce morbidity and mortality. The stages are as follows:
1) Sign in (before anaesthetic induction)
2) Time out (before skin incision)
3) Sign out (before patient leaves theatre)

Surgical Safety Checklist
World Health Organization | Patient Safety

Before induction of anaesthesia
(with at least nurse and anaesthetist)

Has the patient confirmed his/her identity, site, procedure, and consent?
☐ Yes

Is the site marked?
☐ Yes
☐ Not applicable

Is the anaesthesia machine and medication check complete?
☐ Yes

Is the pulse oximeter on the patient and functioning?
☐ Yes

Does the patient have a:
Known allergy?
☐ No
☐ Yes

Difficult airway or aspiration risk?
☐ No
☐ Yes, and equipment/assistance available

Risk of >500ml blood loss (7ml/kg in children)?
☐ No
☐ Yes, and two IVs/central access and fluids planned

Before skin incision
(with nurse, anaesthetist and surgeon)

☐ Confirm all team members have introduced themselves by name and role.

☐ Confirm the patient's name, procedure, and where the incision will be made.

Has antibiotic prophylaxis been given within the last 60 minutes?
☐ Yes
☐ Not applicable

Anticipated Critical Events
To Surgeon:
☐ What are the critical or non-routine steps?
☐ How long will the case take?
☐ What is the anticipated blood loss?

To Anaesthetist:
☐ Are there any patient-specific concerns?

To Nursing Team:
☐ Has sterility (including indicator results) been confirmed?
☐ Are there equipment issues or any concerns?

Is essential imaging displayed?
☐ Yes
☐ Not applicable

Before patient leaves operating room
(with nurse, anaesthetist and surgeon)

Nurse Verbally Confirms:
☐ The name of the procedure
☐ Completion of instrument, sponge and needle counts
☐ Specimen labelling (read specimen labels aloud, including patient name)
☐ Whether there are any equipment problems to be addressed

To Surgeon, Anaesthetist and Nurse:
☐ What are the key concerns for recovery and management of this patient?

This checklist is not intended to be comprehensive. Additions and modifications to fit local practice are encouraged.   Revised 1 / 2009   © WHO, 2009

SURGICAL SKILLS

What are the degrees of wound contamination?

Wound type	Example	Infection rate (%)
Clean	Incision through non-inflamed tissue, GU or GI tract not breached	<2
Clean-contaminated	Entry into a hollow viscous except colon	8-10
Contaminated	Entry into a hollow viscous with spillage or entry into the colon, open fracture or bites	1-20
Dirty	Perforated viscous, traumatic wounds, presence of gross pus	>25

What are the phases of wound healing?

Coagulation: cytokine release causes vasoconstriction, platelet activation and fibrin formation of a haemostatic clot.
Epithelialisation: epithelial cells from the wound edge and stem cells from the basal epithelium migrate beneath the surface of the blood clot and over viable tissue.
Organisation: neutrophils initiate an inflammatory response from cytokine release and macrophage infiltration. This is followed by fibroblast proliferation and angiogenesis. In wounds healing by secondary intention this is referred to as granulation tissue.
Collagen synthesis and remodelling: fibroblasts produce collagen which cross link to form fibrils and fibres. Collagen synthesis gradually declines and remodelling occurs, which is the balance between synthesis and degradation. Cross links increase with density increasing the tensile strength of the wound with type 3 collagen replaced by type 1 collagen.
Maturation: some fibroblasts contain myofibrils that cause wound contraction. Initial scars are red due to underlying vascularity in the proliferative process with time generating a pale scar.

When are wounds left to heal by secondary intention?

– When primary intention is not possible due to excessive epithelium loss
– Contaminated or infected wounds
– When the wound is under tension or would create a tight compartment
– If the wound has broken down

SUMMARY

Removal of a Naevus
• Wash hands, introduce yourself and explain the procedure
• Check site, consent form and wristband
• Check skin anaesthetised
• Mark elliptical incision length 3-4 times compared with width (to gain adequate margins)
• Excise lesion, close and dress wound
• Dispose of sharps safely
• Send specimen for histology, label forms and pot
• Explain post-operative care

TOP TIPS

✚ You may have multiple pieces of equipment at the station. Your knowledge of selecting the correct instrument/blade will be judged. Try and familiarise yourself with as many instruments as possible by being involved with as many operations as possible.

References:
World Health Organisation. 2009. WHO Surgical Safety Checklist. Available URL http://www.who.int/patientsafety/safesurgery/checklist/en/
McCloy R, Thomas B, Weston J. 2012. Handling tissue. *Intercollegiate Basic Surgical Skills Course Participant Handbook.* London. The Royal College of Surgeons of England, pp. 30-31.

SURGICAL SKILLS

2.19 | Scrubbing Up

> **Scenario**
>
> You are about to scrub for an appendicectomy. You will be assessed on your scrubbing, gowning and gloving technique. On entering the station you will find an assistant and UV cream will be used to assess the effectiveness of your technique.

What things do you have to consider before scrubbing up?

– Consider eye protection, masks and hats to cover hair
– Remove any jewellery and watches to ensure you are bare below the elbows
– Wear appropriate footwear e.g. boots if there is a high risk of blood/fluid loss

How do you set up your gown and gloves?

Open gown and gloves carefully to avoid breaching sterility. When unfolding the gown packaging it should be picked at the corners and folded outwards ensuring you grasp the tip only to minimise contact with the contents.

Demonstrate your scrubbing technique.

Set the water temperature and flow rate to avoid splashing and begin by wetting the hands and forearms. Dispense solution into the palm of one hand using the elbow of the other. Apply the lotion to the hands, forearms and elbows ensuring all areas are covered. A nail pick should be used to remove any dirt from beneath the nails, with the bristle end of the nailbrush to clean the nails for the first scrub of the day. The sponge end of the scrubbing brush should be used to help in the application of solution and removal of debris. This should take a total of 4 minutes. The arms are then rinsed from the finger-tips to elbows. The arms should be kept up and in front of you at all times with the hands held up so the water drains from the elbows to prevent dirty water from flowing back towards the hand. This process should be repeated. A final scrub should stop one-third short of the elbow.

Describe your hand washing technique.

Hand washing involves a 7-step technique and are usually found in scrub rooms of theatre. The steps are as follows:
1) Rub your hands with the palms facing each other.
2) Rub the palm of one hand over the dorsum of the other hand and repeat on the other side.
3) Rub your hands with the palms together and your fingers interlaced.
4) Rub the backs of your fingers with the opposite palm and fingers interlocked.
5) Rub the thumb with the opposing hand in rotary movements and repeat on the other side.
6) Rub the palm of each hand with the fingers of the opposite hand.
7) Rub one wrist and arm using the other hand to the elbow and repeat for the other side.

Demonstrate how you dry your hands.

Pick the hand towel from the top of the gown pack and open it fully. Holding one end of the towel, dry one hand through a dabbing motion from the fingers down to the elbow and repeat on the other side with the other towel. Ensure the towel does not touch any unsterile object or part of your body. Dabbing like scrubbing up should be performed in the direction from hand to elbow. The hand holding the towel should not come into contact with the hand being dried.

SURGICAL SKILLS

Describe how you would gown up.

Being careful not to touch the outside of the gown, locate the neck and pick it up so it is orientated the right way up and allow it to unfold. Carefully place your arms in turn through the sleeves and move outwards being mindful of your surroundings so as not to desterilise yourself. Ensure that you don't allow your hands to exit through the cuff of your sleeves. An assistant will tie your gown.

Describe how you glove up.

If you have not pre-selected your gloves and placed them within the unfolded gown pack, request these from your assistant. When double gloving, the inner gloves should be half a size larger than your normal size.
Closed glove technique: keep your hands within your sleeves holding the gown between the fingers and thumb to prevent them from coming out of the sleeve at all times. Open the glove packet and pick up the right glove ensuring the glove cuff remains turned up and place onto your palm with the fingers facing towards you and the thumb facing down. Grip the glove by the bottom cuff from within the sleeve. Using your left hand pull the top cuff over your fingers and slide your hand into the glove. Pulling on the gown at you forearm will help pass the fingers into the glove. Repeat the procedure to don the left glove by placing it with the fingers facing towards you with the thumb of the glove on your own thumb and pull the sleeve over. By orientating the glove packet so that the fingers are already facing you means that you can pick the glove up with thumb of the glove in contact with your thumb and pull over the cuff.

Describe how you would degown.

Gown and gloves are removed in such a way as to avoid contaminating yourself and others in theatre. As an assistant undoes your gown from the back, you should pull the gown off your arms holding it at chest height. You should pull the remainder of the gown off being careful to keep yours arms up infront of you, wrapping it up and finally removing your gloves.

What is the purpose of the first and second wash?

The initial wash removes transient micro-organisms and reduces the level of resident colonising flora. The aim of further washes is to reduce the micro-organism count further.

What patient skin preparations are there?

There are a number of antiseptic solutions. They are applied several times to high risk areas including the perineum, groin and axilla prior to surgery. When prepping patients they should be applied in a circular or sweeping motion, ensuring that it is applied away from the site of surgery to the periphery. Examples include:
Iodine: broad spectrum antiseptic that works against bacteria, spores, fungi and viruses. It is inactivated by blood, pus and faeces.
Chlorhexidine: this has moderate activity against bacteria but poor activity against spores, fungi and viruses. It is inactivated by soap, plastic and pus.
Alcohol: broad spectrum agent with activity against bacteria, but is inactive against spores and fungi.

Define asepsis and antisepsis?

Asepsis: this is the prevention of introducing bacteria into the surgical field
Antisepsis: this is the destruction of pre-existing bacteria in the surgical field.

In what position should you stand in theatre when not engaged in

any activity?

You must keep your back to any dirty equipment and your hands should rest on your chest or above waist height to show others that you are sterile.

What are transient and resident microorganisms?

Transient microorganisms are those that are transferred onto the skin from various surfaces and environmental surfaces. Resident microorganisms are those that are found to naturally inhabit the skin, found in large numbers underneath fingernails and in hair follicles, sweat and sebaceous glands. The aim of scrubbing is to remove resident bacteria from the skin.

What is the difference between disinfection and sterilisation?

Disinfection is the removal of microorganisms whereas sterilisation is the destruction of these organisms.

What is the procedure for changing gloves intra-operatively?

Intra-operatively gloves may require changing due to puncture, contamination or to place orthopaedic implants. There are two ways this may be achieved; firstly an assistant may don the gloves for you where they will hold the glove cuff out being careful not to touch you as you slide your hand in, secondly you may use the closed glove technique to wear your gloves. Either method requires the hands to stay within the sleeves.

SUMMARY

– Scrubbing is the term given to systematically washing the hands and forearms to reduce microorganism counts
– Use a non-touch technique when wearing gloves so not to expose fingers
– Keeps hands above elbows throughout scrubbing technique
– Always work your way down from your fingers to elbows when applying scrub solution, washing and drying
– Be aware of your surroundings when gowning and in theatre

TOP TIPS

Practice, practice, practice!

References:
McCloy R, Thomas B, Weston J. 2012. Basic principles. *Intercollegiate Basic Surgical Skills Course Participant Handbook.* London. The Royal College of Surgeons of England, pp. 7-9.
McCloy R, Thomas B, Weston J. 2012. Appendix A Gloves and surgical handwashing. *Intercollegiate Basic Surgical Skills Course Participant Handbook.* London. The Royal College of Surgeons of England, pp. 69-74.

2.20 Suturing

Scenario

You are the trauma and orthopaedic SHO oncall at a district general hospital and have been called to see a gentleman who has sustained a laceration over his thumb. You are asked to make an assessment and close the wound.

How would you assess this patient as the SHO?

Take a history, examine the patient and order relevant investigations.

History
– Handedness
– Profession
– Mechanism
– Symptoms
– Past medical history
– Medication history including use of anticoagulants/steroids that may affect management
– Allergy and tetnus status
– Smoking status

Examination
– Site of wound and underlying anatomy
– Depth of wound
– Contamination
– Neurovascular and tendon damage
– Soft tissue coverage

Investigations
– Relevant bloods if concern for need for theatre
– Xray for foreign body and associated factors

How would you manage this patient?

I would wash and close the wound under a local anaesthetic ring block using 1% lidocaine, ensuring I have calculated the maximum safe dose. I would maintain an aseptic technique and prep the area with betadine and administer the local anaesthetic. I would ensure the patient could not feel anything before progressing, and I would wash the wound with 1 litre of saline. I would then close the wound with interrupted 3.0 prolene sutures. If the wound was deep and I was concerned about wound edge approximation and tension I may put a deeper layer of 2.0 vicryl sutures. After dressing the wound I would ensure they were covered for tetnus, give a 5-7 day course of antibiotics and advise on follow-up of the wound and removal of sutures.

How would your management be different if there was an associated fracture?

Fractures can be managed conservatively or surgically. An assessment would have to be made according to the fracture pattern including angulation and rotational deformity to determine if surgical treatment is required. It is particularly important to note if there is an associated dislocation or subluxation of involving joints that may also need surgical intervention. It may be possible to treat simple wounds and fracture patterns with no deformity in the Emergency Department but if there is concern of contamination in the

SURGICAL SKILLS

presence of a fracture a thorough wound washout must be conducted in theatre.

What are the basic principles of suturing?

The basic principles of suturing include:
- Avoiding shearing forces by gently advancing the needle through tissue at right angles.
- Avoiding tension by placing sutures at a distance from the edge of the wound that roughly correspond to the thickness of the tissue, with subsequent sutures placed at length of the bite taken. The exception to this where sutures may be placed at varying distances is when suturing fascia or aponeurosis to prevent fibres parting.
- Closure of long wounds by interrupted sutures, to approximate the edges by placing the first stitch in the middle of the wound and successive stitches at a distance half of that length on so on until full closure is complete.
- Avoiding tying sutures under too much tension to prevent cut out and ischaemia.
- Suturing one tissue edge at a time, where it is only permissible to suture both edges at once if they in close proximity to ensure accurate closure.
- Everting skin edges so that the dermis from both sides of the wound are in contact so the wound heals better.
- Allowing enough suture length to be left when sutures are secured and cut to be able to grasp and remove it.

What are the properties of sutures?

Sutures must:
- Be sterile
- Be easy to handle, tie and secure
- Cause minimal tissue reaction
- Maintain tensile strength while tissues are healing
- Be non-allergenic

How can you classify sutures?

Sutures can be classified are according material type, fibre type and absorbability.

Monofilament	Polyfilament
Ethilon	Catgut
PDS	Silk
Prolene	Vicryl
	Vicryl rapide

Absorbable	Non-absorbable
Catgut	Ethilon
PDS	Prolene
Vicryl	Silk
Vicryl rapide	

Natural	Synthetic
Catgut	Ethilon
Silk	PDS
	Prolene

SURGICAL SKILLS

Vicryl	
Vicryl rapide	

Describe memory and tensile strength?

Memory:
This is the sutures ability to return to its original shape after deformation. Sutures with good memory can lead to difficulty in handling and knot tying as it tries to unravel returning to its original shape

Tensile strength:
This is a measure of the time taken for a suture material to lose 70-80% of its initial strength. Absorption occurs enzymatically or through hydrolysis. Absorption time or half-life refers to the time required for the tensile strength to reduce to half of its value. The time that elapses before a suture completely dissolves is referred to as dissolution time.

What are the various suture sizes?

Sutures come in various sizes, the smaller the suture the bigger the size, for example 2 being large and 10.0 being small.

Suture size	Examples
2	Tendon repair Closure of other high tension structures
1 0	Closure of abdominal fascia, joint capsule in hip or knee surgery or deep layers in the back
2.0 3.0	Closure of skin under tension Muscle closure
4.0 5.0	Skin closure Large vessel repair
6.0 7.0	Small vessel repair Facial plastic repair Vascular graft closure eg carotid endarterectomy
8.0 9.0 10.0	Nerve repair Opthalmic surgery

SURGICAL SKILLS

Describe the main types of suturing?

Interrupted suturing:
Multiple single loop of sutures placed through both wound edges and secured with reef knots, which are laid to one side of the wound. The distance of entry and exit points on either side of the tissue should be the same length from the wound edge.

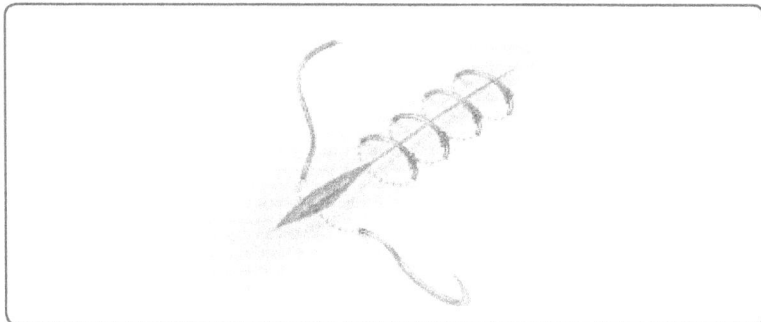

Continuous suturing:
A single suture loop is placed at one end of the wound and secured with a reef knot, with the short end cut. The rest of the suture length is used to close the wound with the next bite taken on the opposite side of the wound obliquely so that when it is passed back onto the side secured with the knot it is at right angles. This is continued until the wound is closed and again secured with a reef knot.

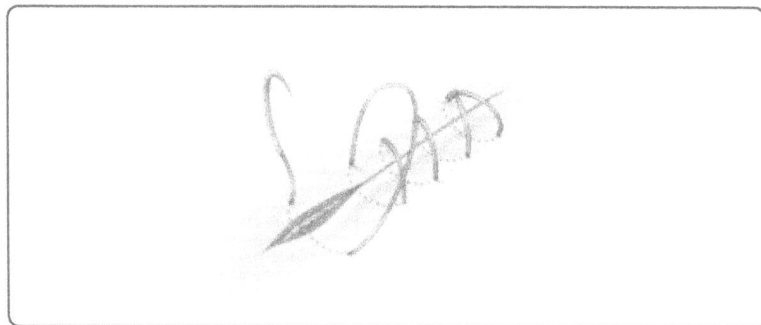

Mattress suturing:
There are two types of mattress suture: vertical and horizontal. In the former a bite is taken as for an interrupted suture, but before tying on the side that the original suture was placed it is looped back through the tissue half way between the exit point and wound edge. It is then passed through the tissue on the other side at the same distance and in the same plane and secured. In horizontal sutures, the first step for interrupted sutures is again deployed but instead of looping back in the same line as vertical sutures a bite is taken in the horizontal plane at a distance similar to the length of the suture loop and then fed back through the tissue to the other side and secured.

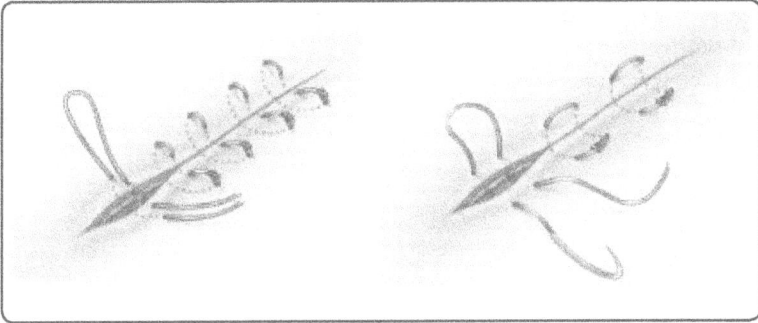

Subcuticular suturing:
This is a continuous snake-like suture, with small bites placed on alternate sides of the wound in the horizontal plane in the subcuticular tissue, which are carefully pulled together.

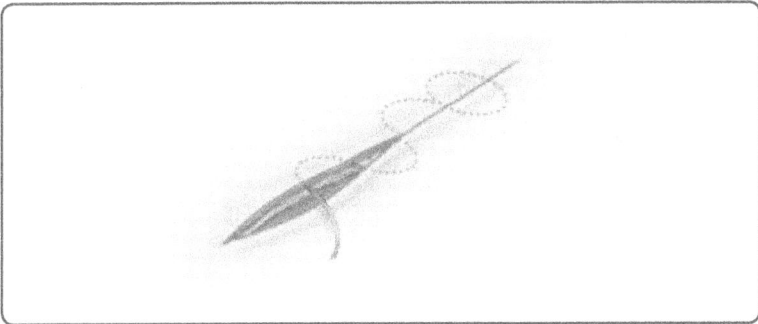

What factors do you have to consider when removing sutures?

When removing sutures, cut flush to the tissue to prevent the exposed length of suture passing through the tissue, which may be contaminated and cause infection. The following is used as a rough guide for the removal of sutures:

Body area	Removal of sutures (days)
Face	4-5
Scalp	6-7
Hands and limb	10
Abdominal wounds	10-20

What other methods of wound closure are there?

– Steristrips
– Glue
– Stapling devices
– Skin clips
– Secondary intention
– Steel wires

SURGICAL SKILLS

What factors do you have to consider when closing wounds and the development of wound infections?

Patient factors	Surgical factors
Elderly thin skin	Excessive wound tension
Malnutrition	Inadequate apposition
Smoking	Poor bloody supply
Diabetes	De-sterility during the procedure/contamination
Steroids	Foreign body
Immunocompromise	Poor planning of incision
Infection	Dead tissue
Hameatoma	
Cardiorespiratory disease	
Anaemia	
Malignancy	
Irradiation	

What is Jenkins rule?

Jenkins rule describes the required surgical suture length for closure of a midline abdominal wound. It is four times the length of the wound when bites are taken 1 cm from the wound edge at 1 cm intervals in the rectus sheath.

What are the different types of needles?

Needles are made up of a tip, body and swage.

Body
– Round bodied: separates tissue as opposed to cutting through it, useful in deeper subcutaneous tissues or anastomoses of blood vessels and bowel, round profile with pointed end
– Cutting: cuts through tough or dense tissue, useful in skin, triangular profile with cutting edge in either the internal or external curve of the needle
Reverse cutting:
Tapercut: combines a cutting tip with a round body

Tip
The tip can be either sharp or blunt.

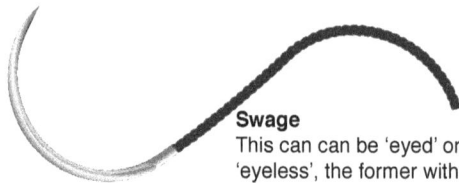

Swage
This can can be 'eyed' or 'eyeless', the former with a hole where the suture is threaded through.

The access to tissue which requires suturing will determine what type of needle you use, therefore smaller operative fields will require a greater needle curvature. Below are the various types of needle curvature:

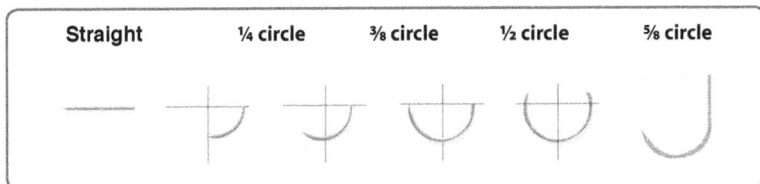

Straight	¼ circle	⅜ circle	½ circle	⅝ circle

Describe how you would perform a tendon repair?

There are a number of ways to repair tendons but the most common method is the modified Kessler repair. The tendon should be handled with care at all times to prevent crushing, which can cause fibrous tissue reaction and tenodesis. The proximal end of the tendon should be sutured first. The entry point of the suture should be ¼ of the way through the cross-section of the cut end towards the length of the tendon. This should pass parallel to the fibres roughly 1.5cm or the diameter of the tendon then exit out from the side. The suture should loop back entering half way through the parallel pass to exit through the cross sectional length on the other side. This should then loop away from the cut end and enter at the level of the initial exit point on the second half of the tendon. The suture is then passed ¼ of the way through that half of the tendon to form a reciprocal longitudinal suture. This procedure is then repeated on the distal end ensuring that the tendon is orientated to carefully match up when reduced, which can be transfixed with the use of needles. The repair is secured with knots that are buried within the cut tendon.

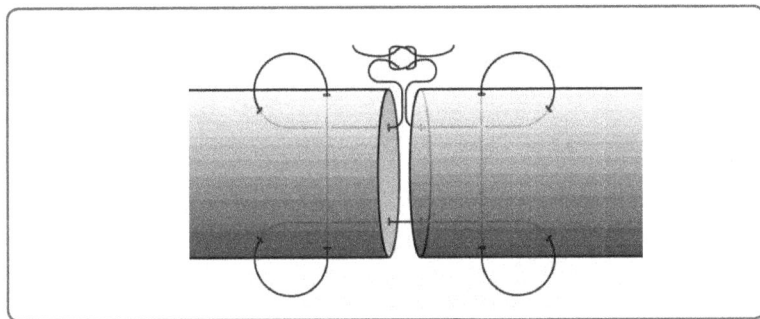

SUMMARY

Suturing is the method of closing wounds and holding tissues together to allow it to repair and heal after injury or surgery. There are a number of different suture types and a number of suturing techniques. A thorough assessment of the wound to be sutured will help select which type and method you use. It is important to appreciate the location of the wound, the steps in wound healing and the factors that can affect it.

TOP TIPS
➕ Practice, practice, practice!

SURGICAL SKILLS

www.ingramcontent.com/pod-product-compliance
Lightning Source LLC
Chambersburg PA
CBHW060448240326
41598CB00088B/4107